P

ANNE AND
DON BYRNE

Psychology

for

Nurses

THEORY AND
PRACTICE

N

First published 1992 by
THE MACMILLAN PRESS LTD
Houndmills, Basingstoke, Hampshire RG21 2XS
and London
Companies and representatives
throughout the world

ISBN 0 333 586 78-6 paperback

A catalogue record for this book is available
from the British Library

Printed in Hong Kong

3077195

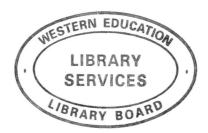

Contents

Preface

Nursing as a science and a profession has made many gains in the past decade or so. Among the most notable of these has been in education, with the transition from an apprenticeship largely under the control of nurse-educators working within the administrative setting of the hospital to tertiary training, where responsibility for the professional training of nurses has been given over to the universities. With this transition, education for nurses has broadened to include a systematic base of the biological and human sciences in addition to the more traditional practical skills training of the past. Nursing has emerged as a profession requiring higher and higher levels of technical expertise. But the practice of nursing also rests squarely with the human sciences; nursing is about people and their lifestyles, about the complex biopsychosocial reasons they become ill, and about the myriad behavioural and emotional responses they show to illness. Psychology is, therefore, a science which is central to the practice of nursing.

There is another side to nursing which is in danger of being overlooked in the present transition. Nursing is, as it always has been, a vocation as well as a profession. Evidence about entry into the profession suggests that nurses are strongly characterized by caring, concern, altruism, idealism, social awareness and a desire to alleviate suffering. They possess, in other words, the personal basis for what psychologists call the *helping relationship*. Large numbers of nurses interacting with and attending to their patients adopt, as if innately, the psychological attributes of an interpersonal relationship which we know, through research, to have enormous therapeutic potential.

Psychology for Nurses came about, then, with all this firmly in mind. The unmistakable transition in nursing education, the identified personal characteristics of those attracted to the profession of nursing, and the centrality of psychology to the broad range of tasks the nurse undertakes all pointed to the need for a textbook which addressed nursing as a helping profession and not simply a set of technical skills. There are, of course, other textbooks which present introductory psychology clearly and scientifically; they are widely used in courses on general psychology and we would not dispute their value for a minute. There are also textbooks on introductory psychology which have been expressly written for the education of trainee nurses, and these too have much to offer. In the main, however, all these texts present psychology in the same way, reviewing the theories and evidence on the classical areas of the science (learning, motivation, cognition, development, personality and so on), but doing so largely out of the applied context in the belief, it seems, that the translation of theories and evidence to the problems of real people will somehow miraculously arise from the simple presentation of the facts.

We have chosen to adopt a different approach. Rather than mirror yet again the 'archetypal' introductory text on psychology, we decided to identify those areas of psychology which are directly relevant to the practice of nursing and to the roles and well-being of the nurse within the broad context of the profession, and to focus on these. In this, we have attempted to integrate psychological theory and evidence with application, presenting sufficient of the former to provide the nurse with a clear understanding and appreciation of basic psychological principles. We have then carefully selected examples from nursing practice to illustrate these principles and demonstrate their immediate relevance to the nurse's clinical work. In this way, we have attempted to go directly to the core of psychology as a contributor to effective nursing practice.

We begin with an overview of contemporary psychological theories and evidence, using the first chapter to acquaint the nurse with the major theoretical and practical areas of psychological enquiry which are likely to have application to nursing practice. In Chapter 2, developing the view that nursing depends for its effectiveness on the establishment of a helping relationship, we seek to explore the nature of helping relationships, closely examining in particular the interpersonal skills which have been established as crucial to these. Chapter 3 extends this to a consideration of practical counselling skills for nurses. Examples of counselling within the nursing role are given, and exercises designed to establish and improve the nurse's counselling skills are presented.

In Chapter 4, the notion of stress and its relationship to the development, course and treatment of physical illness is outlined. The specific role of the nurse in the recognition and management of stress-related conditions in patients under her care is dealt with. Emotions, as psycho-

logical phenomena closely linked with stress, also bear on the development of illness and on recovery from it, and we take the view that nurses
will be primary caregivers in the management of emotional reactions in
their patients. Chapter 5 therefore investigates the principal human
emotions and relates these specifically to the care of patients in the
nursing setting.

In any helping relationship communication is central to success, and
Chapter 6 explores the theories underlying effective communication,
detailing specific demands for communication skills in nursing practice.
The influence of person perception on human interactions in general, and
on the practice of nursing in particular, together with the management
of adaptive and maladaptive perceptual tendencies, is then examined
in Chapter 7. Chapter 8 considers the nature of group structure and
dynamics, and relates this to the specific kinds of groups which nurses
might need to become involved in during the course of their professional
practice. The final chapter looks at the role of psychology in the protection of the nurse herself. This chapter alerts the nurse to the prospect of
burnout, to the recognition of burnout in herself and others, and to the
steps which might be taken for the prevention or management of burnout.

Books presenting overviews of information, for whatever audience,
are necessarily derivative. They draw not only on the original work of
their authors, but on other already published sources of material. This
book follows the same path. In attempting to bring an up to date overview of psychology to a readership of nurses, we have been able to draw
on the knowledge and wisdom contained in many works, and if some are
used often, it is a tribute to their clarity in presenting key psychological
concepts. We acknowledge the value of these sources, and encourage all
readers of *Psychology for Nurses* to explore the references we have
cited. While the basic issues have been discussed thoroughly in this
book, much of the detail, together with the empirical evidence on which
these key concepts are based, may be even better understood by reference to the original material. At the end of each chapter, we have also
provided references to important and informative works not specifically
cited in the text. We have chosen these references because in our view
they add appreciably to an understanding of the subjects covered in each
chapter, and we strongly encourage the reader to explore each area
further by seeking out this additional material.

Of course, we take responsibility for the way the material is put
together in this book, for the opinions and interpretations we derived
from that material, and for any omissions which may be found in its
content. Though we have taken pains to present as contemporary as
possible a collection of material, using current and widely respected
source books and original research papers, the integration of that material and the examples used to enhance its relevance to the practice of
nursing is largely our doing. We took on this task with enthusiasm, and

with a belief, still held, that a knowledge of psychology is central to the theory and practice of nursing, and that without this, the nurse may be constrained from achieving her full potential as a practising professional. We hope this book is able to contribute to this process in some real and material way, and in doing so, is able to enhance the development of what our society holds to be an invaluable profession.

Author's Note

We have used the female gender for all personal pronouns used to refer to nurses throughout this book. We have done this for consistency, and bearing in mind that nursing is still a profession occupied largely by women. We recognize, however, that this situation is changing, and in the past few years, more and more men have sought to enter the profession. This is an occurrence we applaud, and hope that our use of 'she' and 'her' in the text will be taken neither as sexist nor prescriptive of professional expectations in nursing.

1
Elements of Psychology

Psychology is the science of behaviour. It addresses the ways in which organisms behave, or respond to their environments, or react to the myriad stimuli which surround and continually impinge upon them. In more advanced organisms psychology seeks to explain how they perceive, learn, reason, think and feel. Psychology is concerned with the totality of behaviours evident on direct observation. But it also studies the nature of complex environmental stimuli evoking and initiating those behaviours, and the even more complex mechanisms, unobserved but inferred, which are interposed between the stimulus and response, and which mould, mediate, regulate, shape and impose recognizable patterns of individuality on behaviour. From the perspective of the human organism, psychology may be seen as the science most closely and centrally involved with understanding and explaining the adjustment of the individual to the environment. In so far as some individuals fail to adjust, psychology may also be seen as the science of behavioural abnormality or maladaptation. Psychology is, in fact and nature, the complete human science.

This book is concerned with psychology in a very particular context, that of the practice of nursing. The orientation of the book, and the large majority of the examples used in it, will therefore come from human psychology. As we will shortly see, however, psychology has origins in the animal as well as the human sciences. The simple movements of orientation towards a source of light are as much *behaviour* as the complex musings of the scholar. Only the value judgements of the latter, or of his or her species, would make the distinction.

Up to two centuries ago, and for millennia before that, philosophy provided both the structure and the formal discipline for all systematic and objective enquiry about the world around us and about our inter-action with it and with each other. Alchemy, superstition and organized religion all put forward, at one time or another, their own unique and detailed accounts of the origins of the human organism and of its inter-actions with its various environments, that is, its behaviours. These were, however, very strongly dependent on the existence and operation of belief systems, the veracity of which has not stood the test of time. Objective, dispassionate observation of natural phenomena, including the functions and activities of the human organism, and the organization of those observations into categories and ultimately bodies of systematic knowledge was for an extensive period of history the clear province of the philosopher.

With the burgeoning of knowledge across the breadth of human enquiry, the compartmentalization of philosophy was seen to occur. As Morgan & King (1971) have pointed out in their *Introduction to Psychology,* natural philosophy, encompassing investigations into the natural world, both animate and inanimate, became the forerunner of physics, chemistry and biology; moral philosophy, concerned with the problems and issues of contemporary society, preceded the modern social sciences of sociology, politics and economics; and mental philo-sophy, which took account of the thoughts, feelings, motives and actions of individuals, became psychology. Thus, less than a century and a half ago, the publication by Gustav Fechner of *Elemente der Psychophysik,* in 1860, marked the first attempt to collect and present in a single source the evidence then available on the science of the mind. In the follow-ing 20 years psychological laboratories were established in many Euro-pean and North American universities. Their role, to investigate and explain human behaviour, is now taken up by almost every university in the world.

A comparison of some early and more recent definitions of psycho-logy may be instructive in considering its history as an independent science. William James, commonly considered the parent of North American psychology (and brother of the novelist Henry James), wrote in his *Textbook of Psychology,* in 1892:

> The definition of psychology may be best given in the words of Professor Ladd, as the description and explanation of states of consciousness as such. By states of consciousness are meant such things as sensations, desires, emotions, cognitions, reasonings, decisions, volitions and the like. Their 'explanation' must of course include the study of their causes, conditions and immediate consequences, so far as these can be ascertained (p. 1).

Somewhat more succinctly though more sweepingly also, in their 1987 text *Introduction to Psychology,* Atkinson, Atkinson, Smith & Hilgard defined psychology as '. . . the scientific study of behaviour and mental processes' (p. 13).

James' 1892 definition took some trouble to delineate the particular areas of human functioning on which the study of psychology bore. This is not surprising for a definition of a discipline in its infancy, where it is important to establish territorial boundaries and where, perhaps, citing particular areas of interest clarifies the subject matter for the novice, the student or the outsider. The 1987 definition is more broadly sweeping, suggesting a greater confidence in both the subject matter of psychology and its integrity as a discipline. One thing is clear from both definitions: psychology has to do with the entire breadth of mental processes and the activities these direct and regulate. A new word has found its way into the latter definition, however, that of 'scientific'. Indeed, Atkinson *et al.* give a collection of nine definitions of psychology from 1890 to 1981, and six of these use the terms 'science' or 'scientific' to refer to the approach which psychology takes to the understanding and explanation of behaviour. Moreover, the more recent the definition of psychology, the more likely it is to present the view that psychology is a discipline characterized by the application of the scientific method to enquiry into its subject matter, however broad that may be.

Psychology and Scientific Research

Contemporary psychology, then, is *a science*, but what, we might ask, is *science*; what is there about psychology which distinguishes it from, say, a discipline of the humanities (psychology is, after all, largely about people), and what branch of science best summarizes what psychology is about? A brief look at the early history of psychology serves to answer some of these fundamental questions.

As psychology emerged from philosophy as a distinct discipline, the dominant issue concerned the mechanisms responsible for the translation of sensation or experience into action or behaviour, and the dominant method of investigation was introspection. That is, people were asked to reflect on the conscious mental events occurring in themselves between the receipt of a sensation and the initiation of some response to it, and to attempt to report or verbalize these events at some later time. This was very much the approach of early psychologists like Gustav Fechner and Willhelm Wundt, both working in Germany prior to the turn of the century. It represented a major departure from earlier forms of investigation into mental or indeed all other natural phenomena, which relied wholly on external observation of events, detailed recording of those observations, and subsequent (*post hoc*) organization of collected observations into bodies of knowledge. Now, rather than natural observation, investigators deliberately set up situations allowing them some access to the mental events of others under 'controlled' conditions. To be sure, these 'controls' were nowhere near as rigid as those seen in more modern psychological investigations (which we will turn to a little later), but they did allow the experimenter to collect data in a systematic way, free to some extent from the biases inherent in casual and often unguided observation.

We have now introduced a new term, that of *experimenter*, which betrays the nature of this new form of investigation. The early psychologists were, in fact, employing the methodology of experiment. That is, they deliberately created conditions designed to produce mental events (the presentation of a physical stimulus such as a light or sound, the challenge of remembering a sequence of words or numbers and the like) and collected data — the recollections of their subjects' perceptions on what was mentally happening to them, or more accurately, within them, under those conditions, either as they were presented or immediately after. While this method of data collection, that is, introspection, is no longer regarded as an accurate or reliable method for the gathering of psychological information, the beginnings of the experimental method in psychology had far-reaching implications for its development into the twentieth century.

As psychological laboratories grew in number, their reliance on the experimental methodology grew in strength. The earliest investigations centred on the most basic mental processes of perceiving, thinking and reasoning (these may be included under the general and more modern label of *cognition*). That is, psychologists at the turn of the century were most concerned with the ways in which we experience the world and organize the information we gain from those experiences. Just a few years later, however, other psychologists such as James Watson in North America and Ivan Pavlov in Russia developed a keen interest in our use of, and adaptation to, the information we receive from our experience of the world, that is, in our responses to environmental or mental events (we might give this the more modern collective term of *behaviour*). They turned their scientific attention, in other words, to the processes of learning. In this new and developing area, Watson specifically rejected the notion of introspection (indeed, much of the work was done with laboratory animals largely unequipped to report their subjective experiences). Introspection, he claimed, was too subjective a tool to provide valid, reliable and repeatable evidence on psychological phenomena, even if the subject was capable of verbalizing his or her account of the experience. Watson opted, rather, for the more rigidly controlled experiment, where external observations of behaviour (sometimes with the aid of automated recording equipment) took the place of subjective self-report as the principal means of data collection.

In the traditional psychological experiment, the object of the exercise is to collect data which throw some light on a preconceived research question (called an *hypothesis*, which we will define a little later). Two sets of variables are under consideration in any experiment: the *independent variable(s)*, which we wish to hold under control or vary in quite specific ways, in line with the expectations of the research question, and the *dependent variable*, which we expect to vary or alter in accordance with control or change in the independent variable(s). The dependent variable, of course, is that which we observe or measure, and call *data*. We therefore construct a situation in which a collection of observations or measures of the dependent variable are made (data collection) under conditions in which there is systematic and controlled variation in the independent variable(s). Changes in those observations or measures (data) across conditions of the independent variable(s) may then be taken, provided they fulfil certain statistical criteria, to indicate a causal effect of the independent variable(s) on the dependent variable.

Let us make this a little more concrete. Say our research question concerned the capacity of laboratory rats to learn a particular behaviour, such as pressing a small lever in an experimental cage. We were interested to know whether the level of sugar in water (i.e. its sweetness) given as a reward for lever pressing had any effect on the efficiency of the animal to learn. We would then take a colony of laboratory rats, divide them randomly into samples, systematically vary the sugar concentration (sweetness) of the water given to them as reinforcement for their learning task (the independent variable), and take a measure of their learning efficiency (the dependent variable). If we found that rats rewarded with only slightly sweet water learned less efficiently, or less quickly, or forgot their learned behaviour more readily than rats rewarded with very sweet water, and particularly if there was some gradient of effect, such that rats rewarded with moderately sweet water performed somewhere between these two extremes, we could claim evidence of a systematic, experimental and causal effect of the sweetness of reinforcing water on the learning performance of the laboratory rat. This *experimental design* may be seen in Box 1.1.

The construction of experiments need not, of course, be confined to problems as removed from the real world as rats pressing bars. Let us consider an example closer to the focus of this book. Nursing, as we shall see in later chapters such as that on burnout, is a profession carrying with it certain psychological and emotional hazards, many of which are related to the structure of professional organizations within which nurses work. A researcher in nursing policy may, having surveyed the available literature, arrive at the view that level of training and size of hospital have something to do with job satisfaction among nurses. An experiment could therefore be devised and data collected to allow this view to be tested. Subjects would be nurses, but since nurses vary in their levels of training, a large *sample* (ideally, representative of the *population* of nurses from which the sample was drawn) could be subdivided into smaller groups according to level of training (say, single certificate nurses, multiple certificate nurses and nurses with university degrees). Hospitals also vary according to size, and so these groups could be further subdivided according to the size of the hospital in which they work (say, 100 beds or less, 101 to 499 beds, and 500 beds or more). This

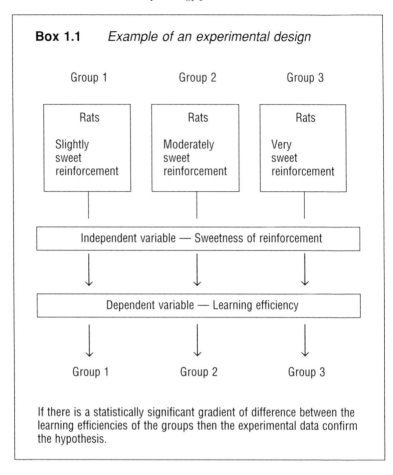

Box 1.1   *Example of an experimental design*

Group 1   Group 2   Group 3

Rats	Rats	Rats
Slightly sweet reinforcement	Moderately sweet reinforcement	Very sweet reinforcement

Independent variable — Sweetness of reinforcement

Dependent variable — Learning efficiency

Group 1   Group 2   Group 3

If there is a statistically significant gradient of difference between the learning efficiencies of the groups then the experimental data confirm the hypothesis.

would provide an experimental design more complex than that outlined in the rat example, because now we are dealing with two independent variables, level of training and hospital size. Having established the experimental design and drawn the samples, some measure of the single dependent variable (job satisfaction) would then be administered, and these data tested for differences between *cells* (a cell being defined by some discrete level on each of the two independent variables, e.g. single certificate, 100 bed hospital, or university degree, 500 bed hospital). This experimental design, and the terms we have introduced to describe its elements, e.g. cells, may be seen more clearly in Box 1.2.

Several things make this experimental design different from the one used in the rat example. First, as we said, it poses a more complex question defined by two independent variables. This raises the possibility of *interaction effects*, in which some unique combination of in-

Box 1.2   *Experimental design to study job satisfaction among nurses*

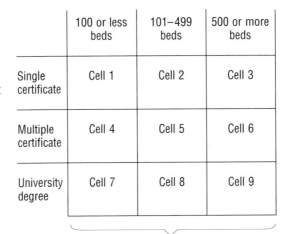

Independent variable 1
(hospital size)

	100 or less beds	101–499 beds	500 or more beds
Single certificate	Cell 1	Cell 2	Cell 3
Multiple certificate	Cell 4	Cell 5	Cell 6
University degree	Cell 7	Cell 8	Cell 9

Independent variable 2 (level of training)

Two independent variables

Dependent variable — Job satisfaction: mean scores in each cell

If there is a statistically significant difference between cells then the evidence supports an effect of independent variable 1 or independent variable 2, or both, on the dependent variable.

dependent variables rather than any single independent variable might be found to explain most variation in the measure of the dependent variable. Second, it is a *natural experiment* rather than a contrived one, in the sense that levels of the independent variables already exist in the real world, and subjects (samples) are chosen because they are already identified by the characteristics of the independent variables rather than having these somehow imposed upon them by the conditions of the experiment. Third, however, the design of a natural experiment does not allow the degree of control which might be found in a contrived experiment, where all possible conditions which might influence variation in the dependent variable are (ideally) eliminated. Thus, some apparently extraneous variable like the subject's age, probably itself associated with level of training, though unmeasured and untested for in the experiment outlined above, might be more responsible for variation in the dependent variable than those independent variables incorporated into the experimental design and measured as part of the experiment.

Despite these potential pitfalls, the natural experiment is a useful and very widely used research strategy in psychological investigation. One further method of psychological investigation, that of *survey research*, needs to be mentioned. This is not an experimental method, in the sense that both dependent and independent variables are measured simultaneously (occasionally, measurement of the independent variables precedes measurement of the dependent variable), and the influence of one upon the other is tested statistically by indices of association. Subjects are not selected to fit into categories of independent variables but are chosen so that they represent the entire range of variation in the independent variables, or as much of it as possible within the limits of sampling. Statistical indices of association allow conclusions as to whether the two variables (independent and dependent) are in any way related to one another.

Thus, in the example given above, of level of training, hospital size and job satisfaction in nursing, one single, large sample of nurses would be drawn (again, representative of the population of nurses from which it came), and measures of each of the independent variables (level of training and hospital size) and the dependent variable (job satisfaction) taken. These measures could then be tested statistically to allow inferences on (1) how much level of training related to job satisfaction, (2) how much hospital size related to job satisfaction, and, using rather more complex and sophisticated statistical procedures, (3) how much some combination of level of training and hospital size related to job satisfaction.

The Theoretical Origins of Psychology

As knowledge in psychology accumulated, its theoretical bases diversified. Distinct schools of psychological enquiry emerged, even in the very early days of the science. Morgan & King (1971) identified the development of five such schools, namely structuralism, functionalism, behaviourism, gestalt psychology and psychoanalysis. We will briefly consider each of these, since they provide some insight into the blooming of psychology from a simple, somewhat concrete science into a multifaceted approach to the understanding of human behaviour.

Structuralism

The preceding development of elemental theories in the physical sciences led to the view, when psychology was still an 'infant' science, that an understanding of the complexities of human behaviour could be built up from the detailed study of the elements of that behaviour. Elements, in structuralism, consisted of sensations perceived by all the sensory modalities (sight, hearing, touch, taste and smell), and of the detailed meanings and interpretations which individuals ascribed to these sensations through the process of introspection. Structuralism attempted to reduce behaviour to its most minute components and then to built up more complex pictures by combinations of elements, just as a chemist might describe the structure of complex molecules by combinations of simpler molecules joined together in predictable and invariant ways. Needless to say, more modern developments in psychology have shown human behaviour to be far too intricate a phenomenon to lend itself to explanation in such concrete terms.

Functionalism

This school held that behaviour and cognitive processes were adaptive, that is, they facilitated individual adjustment to changing environments. In this sense, functionalism bore a close relationship to the Darwinian notion of natural selection, where the capacity to adapt endowed survival value on the individual over others less capable of adaptive change. Functionalism, as opposed to structuralism, viewed behaviours as discrete and complex entities, capable of function in their own right and independent of whatever their elemental structure *might* be. The role of the functionalist in psychology was to investigate both the ways in which basic psychological functions (learning, memory, thinking, etc.) operated, and the manner in which such operations facilitated adaptation to the environment.

Behaviourism

Watson's rejection of introspection as a method of psychological investigation, and its replacement by the controlled experiment, heralded the beginnings of behaviourism, and while both structuralism and functionalism were short-lived influences on psychological theory, behaviourism has survived into the present era. The focus of behaviourism was, quite bluntly, on directly observable actions (behaviours), open to objective measurement and capable of replication under controlled conditions. Pavlov's demonstration that simple physiological responses could be conditioned to appear in a reflex fashion really established the basis for behaviourism. Learning was (and remains) an essential theoretical component of behaviourism, and complex human behaviours were explained in terms of intricate aggregations of more simple, reflex connections (more recent formulations would suggest that this is not a completely satisfactory approach to the explanation of human psychological functioning). Much of the early work used animals as experimental subjects, and though sweeping generalizations were then made from animal to human behaviour, contemporary psychological thought recommends a more cautious and direct approach to the explanation of human behaviour. None the less, behaviourism has had a widespread and significant influence on the theoretical development of psychology, and its influence continues.

Gestalt Psychology

The emphasis of gestalt psychology was on the organization of elements of an experience into a complete perception. Thus, gestalt psychologists were concerned with the ways in which individuals took discrete experiences (a broken line, colours, a series of sounds and the like) and wove these into an overall view of the situation not just made up of the combination of those elements, but also conveying some meaning. Elements of an experience might, for example, only consist of a series of dots, but these, together with their configuration, may convey the overall experience of a circle; so, the individual, when asked what the dots did convey, would be likely to report *a circle* rather than simply *a lot of dots*. This reveals the summarizing principle of gestalt psychology, that 'the whole is more than simply the sum of the parts making it up'. The methodology of gestalt psychology, that of phenomenology (the description and classification of phenomena), at its simplest level is nothing more than the subjective self-report report of experiences, given meaning by the application of a common label.

Psychoanalysis

The advent of Sigmund Freud's work was crucial to the emergence of modern psychology since it shifted the focus away from experience and the processing of information and directed it clearly onto personality. Freud was the first to postulate a comprehensive and systematic account of individual differences in response to environmental demands, by the detailed examination of childhood experiences and the use of these to construct a theory of the direction of adult behaviours. For Freud, the basis of all adult behaviours, normal or abnormal, lay with the adaptation (or otherwise) of the child to interpersonal challenges encountered during clearly and rigidly defined developmental stages occurring in the first five years of life. The methodology of psychoanalysis was far removed from the experimental approach of behaviourism and closer to the introspectionist methods of the structuralists. More than this, however, it relied heavily (and still does, for psychoanalysis, at least as a method of psychotherapy, is alive and well today) on the subjective but 'educated' interpretations of the trained psychoanalyst to give meaning to individual experiences arising as part of dreams, free association and other evocative circumstances. While the essentially interpretive subjectivity of psychoanalysis has been and continues to be criticized for its lack of methodological rigour and the fact that its constructs are not open to direct test under controlled conditions (an experimental approach), its impact on the development of psychology remains, because psychoanalysis, above and before all other theoretical approaches to psychology, sought explanations for the integrated totality of an individual's behaviours, and not isolated examples of these.

In addition to these five schools of psychology, however, an examination of the historical and theoretical background suggests that two further areas of discourse which should be considered. These are humanism and empirical eclecticism.

Humanism

Though arising from psychoanalysis, the humanistic approach to the explanation of human behaviour departs from the rigidly organized structure of the former by viewing behaviour as the emergent consequence of the individual's striving for self-actualization or personal mastery in the face of a sometimes hostile environment. Carl Rogers, to whom the development and great popularity of humanism in psychology may be attributed, believed self-actualization, defined as the inherent tendency of the organism to develop all its capacities in ways which serve to maintain or enhance the organism, to be the primary motivating force for all individuals. Personal experience, as the basis of personal reality, is central to this view, and an overriding need for self-regard or self-worth dominates the individual's search for experiences and for validation of them. When there is conflict between experience and validation, loss of self-regard comes about, and this, in turn, results in symptoms of distress and behavioural maladjustment. The person is at the centre of the humanistic tradition, with all else serving to create and maintain the self-regard so necessary for a healthy psychological existence. Though the data supporting this approach to behavioural explanation is firmly based on the personal experience of the individual (that is, phenomenological), Rogers' work and that of his followers has a strongly empirical tradition, with the quantitative test of hypotheses, largely through the systematic evaluation of their psychotherapeutic applications, being prominent.

Empirical Eclecticism

Few textbooks of psychology make reference to this, yet a century after the beginnings of psychology as a discrete science, it must be recognized that no single theoretical approach to psychology has provided a completely satisfactory and self-contained explanation of human behaviour. Thus, few modern psychologists would espouse a theoretically purist stance to the advancement of knowledge in their science. Most would draw broadly from the diverse wealth of theoretical positions, guided only by the suitability of a particular theoretical approach to the problem at hand and by the empirical respectability of the data they can bring to bear on that problem. Modern psychology draws heavily on an empirical tradition. Contemporary bodies of knowledge in most if not all fields of psychology are developed and consolidated from the results of research studies, themselves undertaken to test hypotheses derived from observation or from earlier, perhaps less well developed theoretical positions. Current applications of psychology are guided both by prevailing theoretical views and by the results of empirical evaluations carried out to examine the effectiveness of psychological strategies applied to the real problems of individuals, groups or communities.

But while most psychologists, theoretical or applied, would nowadays proclaim the primacy of data-based approaches to the explanation of human behaviour, few would restrict their fields of enquiry or of application to single theoretical or conceptual positions. There are, of course, exceptions to this general view. Some social psychologists, for example, continue to believe that the study of social behaviour within the tight confines of the experimental paradigm provides data of sufficient generality to allow useful inferences to be made about human behaviour occurring in the far less rigidly controlled environment of the 'real' world, where a myriad of unanticipated and uncontrolled variables impose themselves upon the individual to shape behaviour in all manner of ways, both obvious and subtle. Some clinical psychologists continue to apply the behaviourist approach rigidly to the treatment of psychological disorders, assuming that all complex human behaviour, normal or abnormal, can ultimately be explained and modified in terms of composites of more simple, learned elements of behaviour, even though the capacity to reason and to interpret experiences places humans at a far higher level of abstraction than the laboratory animal, the study of which has given rise to most behaviourist theories. The large majority of psychologists, however, recognize the fundamental complexity of human behaviour, and as such the fact that control of behaviour by single variables or simple sets of them, no matter whether intrinsic to the individual, occurring within the broader social context of behaviour or encountered during the course of developmental experiences, is practically untenable. By extension, the large majority of psychologists in the late twentieth century, in seeking to explain or to alter human behaviour(s), draw widely from all available and credible theoretical positions, guided above all by the direct and demonstrated suitability and applicability of any theory or theories to the behaviour(s) of immediate interest.

Basic Principles of Psychology

Psychology is not a unified discipline but, as we have stated, takes as its subject matter the whole field of behaviour. Behaviour comes in many forms, is made up of numerous interacting components, and draws on various methodological approaches for its explanation. Thus, the notion that psychology can have *basic principles* is perhaps a little optimistic. None the less, some areas do stand out as distinct fields of enquiry or interest in psychology, either because they represent fundamental building blocks necessary for the integrated understanding of human behaviour (theoretical or experimental areas), because they deal with specific categories of individuals (the young, the old, the maladjusted, for example), or because they address aspects of behaviour which have some self-contained, practical interest (applied areas). The following sections present overviews of the major areas of psychology which are, for one or other of these reasons, distinct, important and central to psychology as a complete discipline.

Biological Psychology

At its most fundamental level, behaviour is organized and regulated by electrophysiological activity within both the central and peripheral nervous systems. Information is received by way of the impact of physical energy of various kinds (light, vibrations in the air or chemical substances, for example) on highly specialized sensory receptors, and transmitted through coded electrical impulses along sensory nerves to the brain. At the level of the brain, information now contained in these electrical codes is filtered, interpreted and given meaning within the extraordinarily complex and little understood circuitry of this crucial organ, and patterns of output representing the individual's response to the now interpreted information are organized and preprogrammed for initiation as observable human behaviours. Electrical impulses conveying the essence of these programs of behaviour are then relayed back through the motor or effector nerves of the peripheral nervous system, to begin and then carefully control through to completion responses which are observably appropriate to the meaning of the incoming messages which set the process in train. These responses, whether simple motor movements like the wave of an arm to deflect an insect, or complex actions like spoken language requiring the integrated involvement of thought, memory, verbal processing and fine motor control, are all behaviours.

Thus, the nervous system, through intricate and exquisitely specific patterns of electrical discharge, based on equally intricate and dynamic processes of chemical synthesis, change and metabolism, takes full charge of behaviour which is, in fact, the most wondrous and infinitely adaptive of all the biological phenomena. Of course, this process does not always work properly or well. While most individuals function within the bounds of physiological normality, some, whether through damage to the anatomical integrity of the nervous system following disease or injury, or disruption to its delicately balanced electrochemical functioning, develop a breakdown of the capacity of the nervous system to perform its many activities. This breakdown may result in a multitude of either obvious or subtle medical symptoms, but it will also be apparent in abnormalities of behaviour, typically of sufficient severity and notability as to indicate to most observers that the individual has ceased to behave in an adaptive or coping fashion.

The centrality of brain–behaviour relationships in the study of modern psychology cannot, therefore, be overlooked. There are, however, some cautions to be observed. While we have seen enormous advances over recent years in techniques of investigation in all of the neurosciences, whether anatomical or physiological, data continue to be either too crude and global (for example, surface electrode electroencephalography) or too minute and specific (for example, electrical discharge patterns of single nerve cells) to allow for the establishment of associations between biology and behaviour which bear directly and usefully on the explanation of the latter. Moreover, much of the precise work in the neurosciences requires invasive experimental procedures, and, in line with obvious ethical constraints, these are restricted to animals or, at best, to human subjects who for independent medical reasons require invasive investigations. This very much limits the extent to which inferences may be drawn regarding the causal influence of brain dysfunctions on complex human behaviours.

Perception

Direct experience with all the infinite phenomena of the external world forms our most immediate pathway to a knowledge of that world. Perception is the study of how we experience the world around us. Sensation lies at the heart of perception. At this level, it is a fundamentally biological process, involving the stimulation of specialized nerve cells (sensory receptors) within sense organs (the eyes or ears, for example) by physical energy, and the transmission of information reflecting this stimulation, by way of coded electrical impulses along sensory nerves, to particular parts of the brain biologically structured to decode this information. The arrival of sensory impulses at crucial brain locations is, however, only the beginning.

Perception is not raw sensation but sensory experience to which meaning has been ascribed. Thus, we do not perceive a physical phenomenon simply as a collected pattern of electrical impulses within some circuit of the brain, but as an object or colour with a name, a sound with a message, a smell with a promise of pleasure (or revulsion) and so on. We perceive sensations as red balloons, gentle music, delicious fragrances, spicy tastes, soft strokes, depressing speech, frightening scenes, revolting odours, nauseating flavours, painful blows and any of a quite infinite array of experiences. At a very simple level, gestalt psychology distinguishes sensation from perception, in that the perceived 'image' is typically more complete than the encoded sensory message relayed neurophysiologically to the brain. A *circular array* of distinct spots of light, for example, is perceived not as an array, but as a *complete circle*. Perception gives a unity and coherence to a sensation which is not strictly inherent in the sensation as a purely physiological event. To do this, perception must involve the equally fundamental psychological mechanisms of cognition, memory and emotion. In its totality, perception incorporates the neurophysiological processing of sensory information, referencing the results of that processed information with past memories of identical or similar sensations, and the attachment of labels and feelings to the present experience.

Cognition

At a very simple level, cognition equates with thinking, and the capacity for conscious, purposeful thought distinguishes humans from all other animals. The philosopher René Descartes, famous for his dictum 'I think therefore I am', considered thought the essence of being. Modern psychologists, however, view cognition as a broad collection of distinct but interrelated mental functions to do with information processing (whether concrete, abstract or symbolic), reasoning, problem solving, decision making, memory, communication, language and imagination. Cognition, in other words, involves the whole range of higher mental functions which allows us to make sense of our environment, adapt to it and modify it, if necessary, to fit our own needs as human beings better.

Cognition is the basis of our unique and individual constructions of the world around us. Through past and continuing experience of the stimulus information constantly surrounding us and impinging onto our consciousness, and the integration of this information into memory, we develop attitudes and beliefs about that world and the experiences it perpetually provides for us. These attitudes and beliefs, couched at times in the form of expectations, act in turn to filter new stimulus information, placing both established and subtly changing interpretations onto that information in a complex, dynamic process which continually updates both the substance and process of our higher mental functioning. We develop 'cognitive maps' of our own, particular worlds, using these not only in the concrete sense of establishing recognition and familiarity with the constant features of the world around us, but also in the more abstract sense of guiding and moulding new responses to stimulus input in novel and unfamiliar territory. In doing so, our cognitive maps are progressively added to, elaborated, refined by the constant exposure to external stimuli, and by constant re-processing of material already in the system, to provide us with an ever more adaptive set of capacities with which to master our environments.

Some psychologists (the influential mental theorist, Spearman, is a good example) have equated cognitive capacity with intelligence. In this equation, an individual's level of intelligence is seen as reflecting the raw capacity of that individual to process and adaptively or constructively use information originating in the external world. Concepts of intelligence have developed somewhat since Spearman's time but it remains fair to say that information-processing capacity sits at the centre of contemporary views of intelligence. Accordingly, it is clear that there are wide individual differences in cognitive capacities. Some individuals, most probably due to fundamentally deficient or inadequate neurological mechanisms arising from genetic endowment, disease or injury (though we cannot overlook the possible role of social and developmental factors, and these will be considered later), will be less able than others to cope with information input and to make good sense and good use of this information once received by the sensory mechanisms. Moreover, individuals will vary in the kinds of cognitive processes they function best in. Some may show greater capacity than others in abstract reasoning but are less capable in verbal or other forms of communication. Some may have substantial capacity in the memory of concrete information but little skill in description requiring novel arrangements of that information. Individual variation in cognition, as in most if not all areas of psychological functioning, is seemingly infinite. Cognitive capacity varies with age. In children, as development of cognitive structures takes place, the capacity for complex reasoning and problem solving may be limited, while in the very old, progressive and inevitable neurological deterioration may result in the substantial loss of most cognitive functions.

Learning

The psychological study of learning deals with the capacity of the individual to benefit from or at least to modify behaviour in the face of experience. At a human level, learning is the process of acquiring knowledge, though in a broader sense, and one which involves animal as well as human behaviour, learning involves a relatively permanent change in behaviour which arises from reinforced practice. The notion of a period of practice is essential to learning, where a series of responses which may at first be 'incorrect' becomes 'correct' through repeated trials and progressive approximation towards the desired behavioural goal, whether through reinforcement or not.

In modern psychology, there have been two paradigms or fundamental processes through which learning is believed to take place. The first of these, attributable to the work of the physiologist Ivan Pavlov, has been labelled *classical conditioning*. The basis for this lies with the automatic association of a stimulus with a response, and the fortuitous pairing of an initially unrelated, second stimulus with the first. Consider the following example. The smell of food elicits the response of salivation in a hungry animal (Pavlov used dogs) previously deprived of food for some time. Thus, a measurable, salivary response may be observed when food is placed before a deprived animal. Since this is entirely physiological in origin, and no learning has yet taken place, the stimulus of food may be called the *unconditioned stimulus* (UCS), and the response of salivation, the *unconditioned response* (UCR). Now, if a quite independent stimulus is paired with the UCS, for example if a bell is rung or a coloured shape is shown each time food is presented, and if this takes place sufficiently often (several trials is usually sufficient with a dog), the presentation of the second stimulus alone eventually serves to elicit the response of salivation. The second, previously independent stimulus now becomes known as the *conditioned stimulus* (CS) and the response, still salivation, having become *conditioned* to the presence of the CS, is now called the *conditioned response* (CR). Thus, through repeated experience, the animal has acquired or learned a new behaviour (it should be said that the learned behaviour disappears, or is *extinguished*, if the UCS of food is not presented every so often to consolidate the learning process). Classical conditioning, of course, is not restricted to animals. Consider yourselves walking repeatedly past your favourite restaurant, smelling the delicious aromas coming from it and feeling your salivary glands surge with anticipatory pleasure, and then some time later, feeling that same surge at the simple sight of the word 'restaurant' in a book or movie. Classical conditioning is, however, largely restricted to responses of a physiological kind.

The second paradigm of learning, known as *operant conditioning* or *instrumental learning*, stems from the seminal work of the psychologist

Burrhus Skinner. The foundations of operant conditioning are reward and punishment or positive and negative reinforcement. These may, in turn, be found in Thorndike's 'Law of Effect' which states that a behaviour followed by pleasurable consequences will be increased in frequency and strength while a behaviour with unpleasurable consequences with be reduced in frequency and strength. The field of operant conditioning, through experimental work largely with animals, has defined in a series of more or less invariant rules the conditions under which reinforced learning will take place. These rules, phrased in their most simple state, in terms of the period or interval between reinforcement and response, and the ratio of responses to reinforcements, are able to predict accurately, at least in laboratory animals, how rapid and how effective a particular learning sequence is likely to be. Learning in the laboratory rat pressing a mechanical bar for the reinforcement of food pellets is strongest, for example, when the reinforcement (food) is given unpredictably and infrequently (a variable interval schedule in Skinnerian terms). Compare that with the behaviour of a person playing a poker machine in which a great deal of 'bar pressing' behaviour is seemingly produced for the unpredictable and infrequent payouts of small rewards.

Clearly, however, it is a large step to generalize from learning research on laboratory animals under highly controlled conditions to the behaviour of humans in far more complex circumstances. Humans are endowed with that distinct feature of cognition, or the capacity to think. We question the frequency and value of reinforcements and the utility of behaviours bringing these about, and we make cognitively based interpretations of the conditions under which learning takes or is supposed to take place. Thus, learning in humans is many times more sophisticated and considerably less predictable than that in animals. Skinner and his close adherents would argue that this is not so; that human learning, though undeniably more complex, is no more than a sophisticated integration of basic learned building blocks, each one established according to precisely the same rules known to govern animal learning. Indeed, complex and global theories of human behaviour have been built up around the notion that all human behaviour is simply grand collections of smaller, more basic units comprising learned responses, put together into broad composites. Several detailed theories of abnormal behaviour rely on relatively simple theories of learning for their origin, and the field of psychotherapy now known as behaviour therapy is based on the belief that abnormal behaviours, however complex, may be eliminated from an individual's behavioural repertoire by simple withdrawal of reinforcement or by the direct application of punishment. Learning is fundamental to the establishment of complex human behaviours, though the rules providing a comprehensive explanation of this process are yet to be fully understood.

Developmental Psychology

This field of psychology deals with those processes concerned with the establishment of psychological functions, from the perception of undifferentiated sensation and the organization and initiation of rudimentary responses in early infancy to the complex and adaptive behaviours required for the adult to survive independently in an equally complex world. Many textbooks of psychology now treat developmental psychology as just part of a continuous process, involving the establishment of new behaviours and their integration into behavioural repertoires of ever increasing complexity during the childhood and adolescent years, the consolidation of these behaviours during the early and middle part of adulthood, and their deterioration, to a greater or lesser degree (depending on the individual), in old age. The term *life-span psychology* has now become an alternative descriptive label for change in psychological functions, whether positive or negative, over the course of a person's lifetime.

In the early years, two types of development, those of *cognitive and intellectual development*, and of *social and personality development*, have attracted considerable psychological study. Cognitive and intellectual development involves the establishment of all those mental capacities discussed above in the section on cognition. As the child develops both physically and neurologically, it establishes a unique concept of the world around it through direct experience and the integration of that experience into more and more sophisticated concepts of reality. At the same time, it develops the capacity to reason, to function with abstract concepts as well as with concrete information, and to deal with symbolic as well as simple oral communications. The psychologist Jean Piaget was responsible for the most systematic and cohesive theory of cognitive development, claiming that this takes place in an invariant sequence of stages, from the purely concrete concept of the environment in early infancy to the capacity to function with abstract concepts in early to middle childhood. Though there has been some debate on the generality of this theory across cultures, it continues to hold considerable credibility among many developmental psychologists and forms the basis for a great deal of contemporary, empirical research in the area. Clearly, there is individual variation in the speed and success with which infants and children pass through the so-called Piagetian stages of cognitive development, and this variation, though not necessarily linked to the Piagetian model, forms the basis for the large amount of current research and practice occurring in the applied specialty of educational psychology.

The development of social behaviour and of personality has been variously explained by two, somewhat conflicting, approaches. Traditionally, the psychoanalytic or psychodynamic theory of Sigmund Freud was seen as the quintessential approach to personality development. This holds that the framework of personality (we will define personality later) which we carry through to adulthood is established in the first five years of life, as we progress through a set of developmental stages which are, like those put forward by Piaget for cognitive development, arranged in an invariant sequence. Experiences which we encounter during each of these stages, very largely to do with the interactions and relationships we have with our parents, allow or impede the flow of *psychic or libidinous energy*, depending on the nature and outcome of those experiences, from the infantile and impulsive *id* to the reality based and adaptive *ego*, and thence to the controlling *superego*. Satisfactory progress through these developmental stages (*oral, oral–sadistic, anal* and *genital*) results in an adaptive balance of libidinous energy between the three divisions of the psyche, and a personality quite able to cope with the complex demands of adult life. Failure to negotiate one or other of these stages successfully produces a personality impaired by a disproportionate distribution of libidinous energy between the three divisions of the psyche and so is dominated by that division, typically the id or the superego, associated with the particular stage of development at the time. Difficulties with the oral stage may, for example, leave the individual with a dominant id and a subsequently impulsive personality, while problems during the anal stage may produce, in adult life, a rigidly compulsive individual dominated by an excessively strong superego.

In more recent times, however, psychologists have found difficulties with this theoretical approach to the explanation of personality, largely because it is not open to empirical test under controlled conditions. Other theories, more closely derived from experimental data than from clinical observation, have supplanted the prominence of the psychodynamic approach, and the social learning theory of Albert Bandura has been foremost among these. This theory, like that of Freud, sees the origins of human behaviour in the early years of childhood, but proposes no invariant set of developmental stages through which the child must pass in order to develop an adult behavioural repertoire. Rather, Bandura suggests a continuous process whereby the child learns new behaviours for its developing repertoire by observing the behaviours of others around it and acquiring or rejecting new behaviours depending on the observed consequences that these have for others. In infancy and early childhood the principal models for observational learning will be the parents; however, as the child becomes more mobile and more capable of physically and cognitively interacting with its world, siblings and others in the household will be observed and their behaviours modelled on. Later still, peers and teachers will enter into the process, as will other individuals, whether personally known to the child or not, whose behaviours and their consequences may be observed (television plays its undeniable role here).

Bandura has set out the characteristics of models which determine the relative strength with which a child will adopt modelled behaviour.

These include the familial or other closeness of the model to the child, the model's status and power in the child's perception and, as we have said, the desirability of the consequences which the child observes resulting from the model's behaviour. The empirical basis for this observational learning approach to development, together with its application as a psychotherapeutic tool in adult life to eliminate maladaptive behaviours and replace them with desired ones, has added substantial credibility to Bandura's contribution to the explanation of behavioural development.

Of course, neither Freud's nor Bandura's approach, nor any other contributing to or stemming from them, give much consideration to the role of genetic inheritance in the development of behaviour. The evidence on genetic determinants of psychological development are not clear, largely because of the great difficulty in conducting studies capable of investigating them in ways allowing unequivocal interpretations of results. It is likely that neurological impairments arising from genetically endowed biological defects determine at least the potentials for and vulnerabilities in behavioural development. The bulk of evidence at present, however, places the development of human behaviour firmly within the control of psychosocial processes occurring after birth and in the early years of life.

Personality

Behaviour varies widely between individuals and across situations. Personality is the process underlying that variation. Personality is that set of guiding principles which determine how an individual will behave in response to the limitless and ever changing circumstances which life creates. There are many views on how personality is structured and equally many theories of how it comes about. Traditional theories, however, consider personality to exist as *type* or *trait*, the two being somewhat complementary concepts. Personality types are made up of groups of individuals all possessing some characteristic or set of characteristics related to their mode of behaviour which distinguishes them from other groups of individuals possessing different sets of characteristics. Though his theory is not now accorded great credence, Sheldon, for example, considered that personality types were closely related to types of body build and stature, with the thin body typically associated with a shy and withdrawn personality, an overweight body with a happy and carefree personality, and a muscular body with an aggressive and competitive personality. Although there is little empirical data to support these observations, the stereotype persists today.

Trait theories of personality postulate the existence of enduring sets of predispositions underlying all human behaviour, accounting for the regularities of individual behaviour and for the behavioural distinctions between individuals. Though different theories have put forward different collections of traits to explain behaviour, all agree that traits are stable within an individual over time and are established very early in the individual's life. Some theorists, for example Hans Eysenck, have argued that personality traits are largely passed on from one generation to another through genetic inheritance, and that within any individual, patterns of personality are determined by fundamental individual differences in neurophysiological activity within the central nervous system. Eysenck's theory proposes, in fact, that all individual personality may be explained by variation along two independent continua of *introversion–extroversion* (which might be loosely seen as outgoingness) and *neuroticism* (instability in the face of stress). He goes on to suggest particular personality types based on possession or absence in the individual of these personality traits. As may be seen in Figure 1.1, the *hysteric* individual is quite distinct from the *dysthymic* individual, in that while both are high on neuroticism, the hysteric is also extraverted while the dysthymic is introverted.

Other trait theorists, for example Raymond Cattell, have put forward more complex trait structures in which up to 35 traits are required in order to account for the breadth of human personality satisfactorily. Whatever the real number, trait theories continue to hold considerable influence in the explanation of personality. Not all agree, however, with the notion that human behaviour is regulated by personality traits invariant over time.

Contemporary approaches such as those of Walter Mischel hold that personality is to a large degree situationally determined. For Mischel, individuals are guided not so much by traits but by *person variables*, developed through social learning, which include *competencies* (funda-

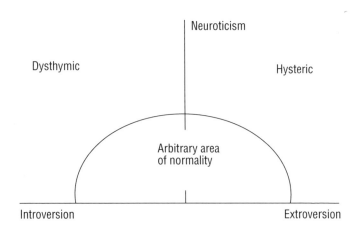

Figure 1.1   *Representation of Eysenck's personality theory*

mental intellectual, social and physical skills), *encoding strategies* (individual perceptions of specific environmental situations), *expectancies* (of what might happen in different situations and of what behaviours are expected), *subjective values* (varying value judgements of situations and of people in them), and *self-regulatory systems and plans* (standards and rules guiding individual responses to specific situations). These may be brought to bear in varying degrees, in an infinite set of combinations, reflecting the unique characteristics of situations calling for behavioural responses. Thus, to invoke the notion of enduring traits of personality acts to limit the individual to a course of action, the narrow scope of which is not confirmed by reality.

Personality theorists differ, too, on how they view the origins of personality. For some, as we have said, genetics plays the strongest part. For most, however, the origins of personality are to be found in the developmental experiences the individual encounters in the years of infancy and early childhood. Whether the theory is based on psychoanalytic concepts or on the social learning approach, developmental experiences involving the young child's interaction with the world around it, and particularly with important people in it, act in a completely logical fashion to mould the building blocks for adult behaviour.

Abnormal Psychology

It will be clear from much we have already said that human behaviour varies, both between individuals and within the same individual but across situations. Behaviours can be and for the most part are adaptive. That is, they contribute to the overall comfort of the fit between the individual and the environment, allowing responses to situational demands which maximize the individual's survival potential and sense of well-being. Some behaviours, however, are inconsistent with adaptation. All individuals show such behaviours at one time or another in their lives. For a few people, maladaptive behaviours come to dominate, either in number or degree. These people are the subject of abnormal psychology.

Broadly defined, abnormal psychology concerns those individuals whose behaviours, thoughts or feelings, of whatever kind, deviate further from statistical norms than are personally comfortable, or than a prevailing set of social and cultural attitudes is prepared to tolerate. Abnormal psychology attends to the description and classification of thoughts, feelings and behaviours which are judged to be abnormal, and to causal explanations of these phenomena, using the broadest range of theoretical and methodological approaches available in psychology at large. It also takes into its field of enquiry the development and evaluation of psychological procedures likely to modify behavioural maladaptation and alleviate psychological distress.

The notion of *deviance* is crucial to abnormal psychology. Abnormal behaviour is deviant behaviour, and in psychology, deviance is first a statistical concept, where normality equates with average. However, while statistics quite adequately copes with the numerical specification of average (simply, the mean value of a set of scores or figures), and while statistics also allows the calculation of numerical indices describing the degree of deviation from the mean, it does not help further in the definition of abnormal psychology, since it does not tell how far a given behaviour must deviate from the mean before it leaves the realm of normality and becomes abnormal.

In deciding when a certain behaviour becomes abnormal, the concept of tolerability must be invoked, and two senses of tolerability are pertinent to the discussion. First, as the definition states, individuals may make their own decisions as to how much of a particular behaviour, thought or feeling is comfortable and, therefore, tolerable. How much anxiety or depression, for example, is tolerable before the individual decides that the bounds of normality have been breached and that help should be sought. Second, and again as stated in the definition, societal and cultural attitudes prevailing at a given time and in a given place may be used by communities or societies to set the limits of tolerance. How far will an individual be allowed to engage in behaviour at odds with the comfort or welfare of the whole community (explicit public sexual behaviour, perhaps, or gross interference with the rights of others) before the community, or delegated representatives of it, decide that tolerance has been exceeded, and act to restrict the free movement of the offending individual in that community. While these are questions as much to do with philosophical and moral as with psychological considerations, they underscore the view that decisions regarding psychological abnormality are ultimately subjective ones, most often made by individuals exercising, perhaps arbitrarily, their own constructions of the world.

It follows from this that what is considered to occupy the field of abnormal psychology will not necessarily be consistent over time or place. Attitudes of tolerance in relation to particular behaviours will change over the course of history, in line with social and political changes, and these will bear strongly on what, at any given time, will be judged abnormal. The same may be said for cross-cultural differences in attitudes towards human behaviours. Abnormal psychology, therefore, will always be a relative field of scientific enquiry, seeking descriptions and explanations of abnormal behaviours, but recognizing the dependence of these on time and place. To the extent that most studies of abnormal behaviour are conducted within the largely similar settings of Western, urbanized societies, this does not pose a great problem, though it recommends caution against broad generalizations of statements of absolute truth in abnormal psychology.

Social Psychology

All behaviour occurs in some context. Since the large majority of people live in social groups of one kind or another, behaviour typically occurs within a social context. Social psychology addresses the ways in which the social context influences behaviour, and conversely, the ways in which individual behaviour acts to influence the social circumstances surrounding it. Gordon Allport, a prominent theorist in the area, said of social psychology that it concerned the explanation of how thinking, feeling or behaving in any individual is influenced by the presence of any other individual or group.

Social psychology focuses clearly on the individual (as opposed to sociology, which takes the broader society as its point of reference) and attempts, through survey or experiment, to discover what elements of behaviour are most influenced by social context, and how that influence comes about. Social psychologists have applied the term *social behaviour* to any individual behaviour which has social elements or social consequences. More technically, however, it has come to refer to group behaviour, in which behaviour appearing in a group setting is controlled and moulded by the characteristics of the group and by the interchange between the individual and other members of the group. Thus, the behaviour itself is not the only focus of study; the characteristics of the group, its structure and size, the reason for its existence, the functions it performs for its members, the values its members place on membership of the group and so on are also studied.

The range of issues and areas addressed by social psychology, therefore, is extensive. Since the social context of behaviours is all pervasive, and there is substantial potential for social influence on a multitude of individual behaviours, the central role of social psychology in the broad explanation of behaviour is undisputed. What is in dispute, particularly among social psychologists, is the methodology used when studying social influences on behaviour. Experimental social psychology holds that social influences on behaviour may be understood by conducting experimental studies of small samples, where the social context is controlled or manipulated in (hopefully) known ways, and the effect on consequent behaviours is observed, recorded and quantified. Such studies follow much the same experimental designs as those discussed earlier in this chapter. The value of such studies lies in the degree of control which may be brought to bear on the social context. Their disadvantage is that they may be so highly controlled that the social conditions created bear little resemblance to reality, so severely limiting the extent to which the findings can be generalized to daily, social behaviour.

As an alternative, many studies of social behaviour are conducted in the 'real world', by selecting (usually large) samples of individuals living and functioning within already existing, though certainly com-

plex, social situations over which there is little or no control, but which
are totally real. Individuals in such situations may then be observed, and
their behaviours recorded and quantified, or they can be asked specific
questions about present or anticipated behaviours, as well as about
attitudes, beliefs, expectations regarding the behaviours of others in the
same or similar situations, and so on. The disadvantage of this approach,
which usually relies on the collection of data by self-report questionnaire, lies with the possibility that individuals may not report what they
are actually doing, thinking or feeling, but what they believe the researcher, or society at large, expects them to be doing, thinking or
feeling. The operation of what social psychologists call *social desirability* may, in fact, bias the nature of the data collected and, therefore,
the kinds of conclusions which the social psychologist draws from those
data.

Applied Psychology

For at least two reasons, it is not totally accurate to speak of applied
psychology as a single category, first because most areas of psychological enquiry have applications, and second because the applications of
psychology are extraordinarily diverse. Areas of applied psychology are
not usually identified by their approach (for example, applications of
learning theory) but by the field of application they address. It is well
beyond the scope of this chapter to provide a detailed account of each of
these; however, reference to four of the most central and widely practised fields of application should serve to illustrate the remarkable range
of human problems, to which psychology is able to contribute solutions.

Educational psychology, drawing largely on the theories of developmental psychology, learning and personality, addresses the processes of
education and the capacity of the individual to benefit from these. The
practice of educational psychology includes the application of psychological principles to the understanding of complex human learning and
the ways in which the presentation of information might influence this,
the development and evaluation of teaching methods, and the assessment
of individuals of all age groups so as to guide them into educational areas
and levels most likely to suit their capabilities and needs.

Clinical psychology, which has its theoretical origins in the study of
personality and abnormal psychology, as well as, to an extent, learning
and cognition, focuses on the assessment and treatment of psychological
disorders. In this sense, it is closely related to the medical speciality of
psychiatry, though clinical psychologists are not qualified to prescribe
medication, and commonly take an approach to assessment and treatment based on behavioural or learning principles rather than on
psychodynamic or psychoanalytic ones. In recent times, behavioural
medicine and health psychology, which apply psychological principles

to the explanation, diagnosis and treatment of physical illness, have developed as off-shoots of clinical psychology.

Industrial/organizational psychology covers a wide range of applications relevant to the uses of psychology in the occupational setting. Deriving from many areas of psychology, but largely from social psychology, personality and cognitive psychology, the occupational applications of psychology range from the assessment of individuals in order to facilitate occupational placement to the assessment of occupational environments so as to diagnose difficulties in occupational adjustment. Industrial/organizational psychologists advise on work efficiency both from the individual perspective and that of the occupational environment. They consider the structure and function of organizations, so that they are able to advise on the modification of these to improve work efficiency and reduce occupational stress, and they examine the interpersonal dynamics and processes within occupational settings, so as to maximize the capacity of those in positions of control to manage better the activities of those working for them.

Ergonomics, a very special area of industrial/organizational psychology, based closely on the experimental psychological study of information processing and human response mechanisms, specifically examines the fit between people and equipment. It addresses the design of furniture in a variety of occupational settings in order to reduce skeletal muscle strain, the structure and layout of gauges and instruments in complex displays of information in order to improve the accuracy of readings, the structure and placement of controls in order to reduce error, and a multitude of other functions to do with the physical settings in which occupations are carried out. Occupational/organizational psychology, in all its facets, has much to do with the related discipline of occupational health.

As we have seen, then, the applications of psychology to the solution of human problems is diverse. The underlying theories of psychology lend themselves to considerable application, and the effectiveness of those applications has been amply demonstrated for a wide range of areas and issues. In effect, of course, this simply underscores the breadth and pervasiveness of the science of psychology which definitions, given earlier in this chapter, make clear.

Relating Psychology to Nursing Practice

In its most rudimentary form, the practice of nursing involves the application of medical science to the management of people with physical illness. The technical procedures of nursing can be competently accomplished provided nurses have at their disposal the requisite medical knowledge necessary to attend safely to the physical needs of their patients. They can administer medication, monitor an ECG readout, set up an intravenous drip or change a surgical dressing without recognizing that the subject of their attentions is anything other than a more or less dysfunctional collection of cells organized in highly complex ways to resemble a human being. But nurses cannot talk to patients, enquire about the presence or frequency or severity of their symptoms, respond to their questions, attend to and alleviate their pain and distress, reassure them of their progress, calm them in their anxiety or be with them as they face death with anger or grief, without recognizing that patients are more than the mere external evidence of their biological disorders. Nurses cannot talk with families and friends waiting for news, or expressing fears for their loved ones, without realizing that patients are not just biological individuals, but people existing in complex social worlds, interacting in the most intricate and interpersonally intimate ways with other people, depending on them, and being themselves dependent. Nursing is, therefore, far more than the application of a technically sophisticated biological science. Without understanding the person as well as the biology, the nurse will inevitably ignore a sizeable part of the patient. The study of psychology is central to the practice of nursing in at least four major ways.

First, as we will see in later chapters, psychological factors play crucial roles in the development and course of many illnesses, and in the processes of recovery from them. Stress, which is now seen to play a causal, contributory part in the formation of pathology of many kinds and in the onset of various acute illnesses, is fundamentally a psycho-logical construct, drawing for its explanation on theories of cognition, learning and social psychology. There is now a body of thought in medicine which holds that we no longer question whether or not stress plays a role in the onset of any illness, but just how much of a role stress plays, either for the illness category or for the person who is ill. It is estimated that between 50% and 70% of all people who consult a medical practitioner, even with conspicuously physical symptoms, do so because of underlying psychological reasons and motivations. Indeed, the psychology of the individual is instrumental in determining whether or not a person experiencing symptoms of physical pain or distress, whatever these are, will decide to consult a doctor or seek other medical attention. From another perspective, many individuals nowadays, either through ignorance or lack of care, engage in behaviours which constitute health risks. Poor eating habits, cigarette smoking, excessive alcohol consumption, unsafe driving, drug abuse, unprotected casual sexual inter-course, lack of exercise, failure to comply with prescribed medication or other treatments, and many more, are all clear-cut human behaviours, developed and regulated by fundamental psychological processes but with profound implications for human health and illness. Without under-standing the psychology of illness risk, of the development of physical pathology, and of symptom onset, recognition and reporting, nurses will only ever understand a fraction of illness itself.

Second, nurses must deal not just with the management of physical pathology and its external signs and symptoms, but also with the patients' unique and individual reactions to illness. Illness typically involves pain and discomfort and brings with it uncertainty and anxiety. It may foreshadow protracted physical disability or threaten life itself, and may bring about long financial and personal hardship. Even the medical processes involved in saving life and alleviating physical suffering are likely, in many instances, to be painful, distressing and frightening. Individuals have varied reactions to the entire process of illness. They may become anxious, angry, depressed, uncooperative, uncommunicative, depersonalized, irritable, withdrawn, shallow or abusive; they may regress to childlike states of behaviour or they may become detached from reality in a frankly psychotic manner. All these reactions may be seen to arise from the generalized experience of *distress*. Nor can these be viewed as isolated and acute reactions to illness, difficult at the time but most likely transitory. Responses to illness (we will discuss them as *illness behaviours* in later chapters) can have powerful influences on the course and progress of recovery and rehabilitation following acute illness episodes. It is nurses who are most likely to be closest to the patient during the whole course of illness, and it is nurses, therefore, who are most likely to observe and to have to manage these varied and difficult but common and inevitable reactions. Nurses' skills in observing, listening, empathizing, communicating and caring are as crucial as their skills in medical technology, and their understanding of responses to illness and of their psychological origins and controls, with all their implications for recovery and for future illness, is crucial to total patient care. Failure to appreciate this can only lead to patient care which is incomplete.

Third, as soon as nurses engage in the interpersonal interaction that forms the setting for patient care, they have entered into the 'system'. That is, they have become part of a complex social psychological system comprising the patient, the patient's immediate significant others, medical and paramedical staff in varying levels of power and authority, and of course, themselves. Nurses cannot be isolated and external individuals, operating free from the total psychological context of nursing care. Nor can they expect that their own role, attitudes, behaviours and responses to the situation of patient care will not have their own unique effects on the operation of that social psychological system. Nurses, like all participants in the system, have a *dynamic* and *reactive* role; that is, whatever they do, however they act, whatever their attitudes and behaviours towards the patient, and towards others in the system, these will feed back into the system to alter, whether conspicuously or subtly, the ways in which it operates. This has clear implications for patient care and for the ways in which the patient will perceive and respond to that care. As a consequence, it may bear strongly on the patient's sense of well-being and emotional state and, through well understood mechanisms of illness behaviour and stress, on the rate and success of patient recovery and rehabilitation.

Finally, nurses must understand that they, too, are individuals whose behaviours, thoughts, attitudes and feelings are all governed by the same psychological mechanisms as those of their patients. Like all human beings, nurses will have interests, needs, fears, concerns, hopes, wishes, feelings of inadequacy and distress as well as of success and happiness, emotional limitations, uncertainties, ambitions and a desire to achieve, both for them and for their patients. Nurses are neither mere technicians nor mechanics; they exercise extraordinary technical skill, but do so within a context of interpersonal interaction demanding, as well, the highest possible skills as people. Indeed, research suggests that many nurses choose their profession because they already possess great 'people' skills and a compelling desire to use these skills for the greater benefit of others. In doing so, however, they must recognize that the exercise of such skills may involve personal cost, particularly if they do not simultaneously understand the psychology of patient care and of the structures and organizations in which this takes place. Psychology is central to all these things. It explains behaviour in context, whatever the individual or the setting, and for the nurse, such knowledge, at the very least, facilitates personal survival in what is one of the most demanding of all the professions.

Summary

In this chapter an attempt has been made to describe and illustrate psychology as a human science. First, psychology was defined; it was argued that psychology refers to the study of behaviour and mental processes and is essentially a discipline dominated by the application of the scientific method. Second, the experimental model of psychology was explored in some detail. Third, seven schools of psychology were considered (namely, structuralism, functionalism, behaviourism, gestalt psychology, psychoanalysis, humanism and empirical eclecticism) and their various contributions to the understanding of human behaviour analysed. Fourth, the basic guiding principles of psychology were considered — only those areas which were seen to have made a distinct and important contribution to the study of human behaviour were presented, viz., biological psychology, perception, cognition, learning, developmental psychology, personality, abnormal psychology, social psychology and applied psychology. Finally, an attempt was made to relate the basic principles of psychology to nursing practice.

The remainder of this book sets out to discuss and explain the core roles of psychology in the practice of nursing.

References/Reading List

Atkinson, R.L., Atkinson, R.C., Smith, E.E. & Hilgard, E.R. (1987). *Introduction to Psychology*. San Diego: Harcourt Brace Jovanovich.

Boring, E.G. (1950). *A History of Experimental Psychology*. Englewood Cliffs, New Jersey: Prentice-Hall.

Cohen, J. & Clark, J.H. (1979). *Medicine, Mind and Man: An Introduction to Psychology for Students of Medicine and Allied Professions*. San Francisco: W.H. Freeman & Company.

Deaux, K. & Wrightsman, L.S. (1988). *Social Psychology*. Pacific Grove, California: Brooks/Cole.

Hall, J. (1982). *Psychology for Nurses and Health Visitors*. London: Macmillan.

Heaven, P.C.L. & Callan, V.J. (eds) (1990). *Adolescence: An Australian Perspective*. Sydney: Harcourt Brace Jovanovich.

Hetherington, E.M. & Parke, R.D. (1988). *Child Psychology: A Contemporary Viewpoint*. New York: McGraw-Hill.

Hilgard, E.R., Atkinson, R.C. & Atkinson, R.L. (1975). *Introduction to Psychology*. New York: Harcourt Brace Jovanovich.

Hine, F.R., Carson, R.C., Maddox, G.L., Thompson, R.J. & Williams, R.B. (1983). *Introduction to Behavioral Science in Medicine*. New York: Springer-Verlag.

Hoyenga, K.B. & Hoyenga, K.T. (1988). *Psychobiology: The Neuron and Behavior*. Pacific Grove, California: Brooks/Cole.

James, W. (1892). *Textbook of Psychology*. London: Macmillan.

Kristal, L. (ed.) (1982). *The ABC of Psychology*. Middlesex: Penguin.

McGhie, A. (1986). *Psychology as Applied to Nursing*. Edinburgh: Churchill Livingstone.

Marzillier, J.S. & Hall, J. (eds) (1987). *What is Clinical Psychology?* Oxford: Oxford University Press.

Morgan, C.T. & King, R.A. (1971). *Introduction to Psychology*. New York: McGraw-Hill.

Nixon, M. (ed.) (1984). *Issues in Psychological Practice*. Melbourne: Longman Cheshire.

Reber, A.S. (1985). *Dictionary of Psychology*. New York: Penguin.

Sarason, I.G. & Sarason, B.R. (1989). *Abnormal Psychology*. Englewood Cliffs, New Jersey: Prentice-Hall.

Watson, R.I. (1971). *The Great Psychologists*. Philadelphia: J.P. Lippincott Co.

2
Nursing as a Helping Relationship

At its most fundamental level the practice of nursing involves the intense and some times deeply personal interaction between two individuals, the one being defined by the characteristics of suffering and dependency and the other by the attributes of helping, caring and healing. Much of what a nurse does in her professional role involves the use of technology to relieve suffering, alleviate symptoms and bring about with all possible haste the processes of recovery and so enable the patient to return to his or her normal life. In this role the interaction between the nurse and patient is very much a unidirectional one in which the nurse assumes the position of the authoritative professional whose function is to apply the techniques of treatment and healing, and to lead the patient with competence and confidence through to the point where the relationship is no longer necessary.

This view of nursing, which relies very much for its orientation on expectations of technical skill and an authoritarian view of communication, cannot be denied. In a setting in which the use of knowledge-based strategies and procedures is emphasized and, it could be argued, essential, the pattern of the interaction between nurse and patient is, to a degree, already laid down. This pattern of interaction, defined by the roles of the leader and the led, is of clear importance in some aspects of nursing practice. From a broader perspective, however, it is equally clear that the interaction between nurse and patient is bidirectional; that is, the interaction involves a two-way communication between nurse and patient which transcends the limitations surrounding the mere application of technical strategies and manipulations. In many respects, the interaction between the nurse and the patient is as much a helping relationship as it is a medium for the patient's passive receipt of therapeutic acts.

This multifunctional view of the nurse–patient interaction has parallels in other branches of medicine. While medicine has been seen throughout history as a science or a technology in which the healer (the physician) exerts a healing influence by means of the application of acts and rituals based on professed and accepted technical expertise, it has in recent times come to be recognized that the effectiveness of this healing influence is modified and regulated by the nature of the relationship between the physician and the patient (Gordon, 1976). There is now much evidence from the research literature to support the view that the most effective healer is that person who first establishes a close, confiding and trusting human relationship with the person who is to be the recipient of the healing acts (Stone, Cohen & Adler, 1979). Thus, too, in nursing, it will be seen that the most effective nurses are those who have developed a capacity to enter into a particular human relationship with their patients.

That nursing involves a specialized human helping relationship cannot be denied. This relationship has as its core a number of fundamental principles closely akin to the notion of psychotherapy. While psychotherapy has been variously defined by many people, perhaps the most cogent and personal definition comes from the psychotherapist Frank (1961) who, in his book *Persuasion and Healing*, considered psychotherapy to involve a specialized human helping relationship which met the following three criteria. It involved:

1. A trained socially sanctioned healer whose healing powers are accepted by the sufferer and by his or her social group or an important segment of it.
2. A sufferer who seeks relief from the healer.
3. A circumscribed, more or less structured series of contacts between the healer and the sufferer through which the healer, often with the aid of the group, tries to produce certain changes in the sufferer's emotional state, attitudes and behaviour. All concerned believe these changes will help him. Although physical and chemical adjuncts may be used, the healing influence is primarily exercised by words, acts and rituals in which the sufferer, healer and — if there is one — group, participate jointly.

While this definition of psychotherapy is both broad and general, it encompasses the very essence of psychotherapy as a process, the object of which is healing and the substance of which is defined by roles and relationships. It may be seen from this definition that many forms of human interaction fulfil the criteria for psychotherapy, and that this process extends far beyond the traditional boundaries in which psychotherapy is seen to be the exclusive province of the psychiatrist or clinical psychologist. In a very real sense the interaction which nurses have with their patients may be considered to be as much psychotherapeutic as the more typical view of the psychoanalyst. Psychotherapy is the practice of using this specialized helping relationship to define problems in the patient's personal life, to treat symptoms and, at its best, to help the patient live in ways that better satisfy the enduring needs for affection and mastery (U'Ren, 1980). A great many forms of human interaction have taken on the guise of psychotherapy and some have gone so far as to establish around them some sort of theory which distinguishes one from the other and which guides the practice of the art.

An exhaustive listing of the different forms and schools of psychotherapy would be a time-consuming exercise and is not the purpose of this chapter. A number of excellent texts (see, for example, Prochaska, 1979, or Gilliland, James, Roberts & Bowman, 1984) will provide useful information on the numerous schools of psychotherapy to which the psychotherapist may look for guidance and direction. An examination of the essential characteristics of the broad range of psychotherapeutic schools, however, indicates a degree of variation in the extent to which the human relationship itself acts to influence the process of healing. One major group of approaches to psychotherapy, that which is called humanistic or existential-humanistic, has placed greatest emphasis on the role of the person as director of his or her own life, and regards the role of the helping relationship as a facilitator to that process. Humanistic approaches to psychotherapy view the individual's personality as being in a continual state of growth and change; the individual does not possess a fixed self or character structure or identity but is seen rather as an 'open system', continually interacting with the environment, taking in information, integrating that information with data already in the system and changing in a creative way in response to the continual influx and adaptation to information (Bohart & Todd, 1988). In this chapter we will propose that humanistic approaches to helping relationships provide the strongest and most pertinent theoretical perspective for the examination of the helping relationship in nursing practice. It will be shown that in a multitude of ways, the nurse takes on the role of helper (or, in therapeutic terms, the therapist) while the patient is the recipient of that help (in therapeutic terms, the client), and that the relationship which arises from this interaction exerts a powerful influence on the process of healing. In this way the helping relationship evident in the nurse–patient interaction will be shown to have substantial parallels with that of the therapist–client relationship in the context of humanistic psychotherapy.

A number of schools of psychotherapy have claimed general membership of the humanistic orientation. The school of gestalt psychotherapy, which originated with the work of Frederick Perls (1951), is very much based on the notion that psychotherapy is a fundamental process of human growth whereby the individual, in interaction with the therapist, learns to become fully aware of his or her current existence and to adapt to it. The existentialist approach, which has its roots in the existential philosophies of Heidegger and Kierkegaard, is best exemplified in the work of Rollo May (1961). This approach does not emphasize particular techniques in psychotherapy but rather defines the goal of the therapist as being to develop an understanding of the patient as a unique being and use this understanding to bring about insights within the patient regarding his or her own patterns of adaptation and coping. Both these approaches, while they have attracted their own unique and considerable followings, none the less rely on an unquestioned acceptance by the practitioner, and indeed the client, of rather obscure theoretical foundations which to the uninitiated may be difficult to understand.

However, by far and away the most widespread and accepted of the humanistic approaches to psychotherapy is that deriving from the work of the psychologist Carl Rogers. This work has achieved enormous recognition since its beginnings 40 or more years ago, both for the breadth and simplicity of its concepts and for the documented benefits which it appears to bring to those in distress. The therapeutic approach which we will specifically focus on in this chapter will, therefore, be the *client-centred approach* of Rogers.

Rogerian or Client-centred Psychotherapy

The client-centred approach originated with Carl Rogers in the early 1940s and is first spelled out in his book *Counselling and Psychotherapy* (1942). This work was considered a landmark in the evolution of psychotherapeutic thought and practice. Client-centred psychotherapy or counselling has been a continually growing and changing theoretical system. It was originally known as non-directive counselling, since its approach was to allow the patient or client complete freedom to make his or her own decisions in therapy, to determine the direction of therapy and to regulate the pace with which therapeutic change occurred. All this implies that the focus of attention is not so much on the therapist as on the client, and in later years the therapy became known as person-centred or client-centred counselling. The change of name in recent years from client-centred to person-centred reflects Rogers' personal concern that his approach should be applied to many areas of life beside those involving the psychotherapeutic context alone (Bohart & Todd, 1988). Rogers' approach is, however, still most commonly referred to as client-centred, and therefore this term will be adopted here, with the recognition that it refers to a far wider range of helping relationships than those simply entailed in psychotherapy.

Basic to Rogers' client-centred approach is the belief that all humanity has one single motivating force, this being a tendency towards self-actualization. Rogers defines the actualizing tendency as the inherent predisposition of the individual to develop all his or her capabilities in ways which serve to maintain or to enhance individual integrity, adaptation and well-being (Prochaska, 1979). In order to attain self-actualization the person must have freedom of movement to grow and access to conditions which nurture growth. The fundamental concept of client-centred relationships is that the person in the helping relationship must respect and facilitate the self-propelled growth process in the client. This notion is based on two premises:

1. that there are many possible realities and that no one individual is in a position to judge another's reality; and
2. that if the personal reality of an individual is respected by others and a basic trust is demonstrated towards that person, then a self-propelled growth process will move in a positive and life-affirming direction (Bohart & Todd, 1988).

From the humanistic perspective, Rogers saw the actualizing tendency as bringing people towards each other rather than driving them against each other (Prochaska, 1979). The helping relationship, according to Rogers, involves a process whereby the individual's ability to refer directly to what is experienced as true and meaningful for him or her is restored. This process occurs primarily through self-acceptance. If clients can adopt a non-judgemental self-accepting attitude towards themselves then they can learn to tune into their experiential sense of the world around them and of events in their environment.

In the process of helping, then, the helper must create an environment in which the client is able to focus on his or her own experience and to use the realization of that experience to adapt to the environment and so to grow as a person. By implication, Rogers believes that this personal growth will result in the resolution of personal problems and the capacity to deal more adequately with challenges and problems which might arise at some future time.

The nurse's professional activities are punctuated by encounters with people who are experiencing problems of a moderate or serious magnitude. Illness carries with it the experience of pain and suffering, the threat of incapacity or death and the need for both emotional and material adaptation in the face of prolonged sickness. There is also the impact of illness on relationships with significant others in the patient's life, along with the possibility of social and material hardship and the inevitable challenge to the patient's self-image of physical and emotional integrity. With few exceptions, the nurse is in a unique position to deal with these difficulties since it is the nurse who is most likely to be in immediate and primary contact with the patient. It is the nurse who is most likely to be trusted with the patient's feelings and experiences during times of illness and it is the nurse to whom the patient looks most often for immediate help and caring. Therefore, it is the nurse who is most likely to be able to use the principles set out by Rogers in a manner which allows the patient to focus on his or her experiences and to use that process to achieve self-growth and to resolve the immediate distress of illness. It is not suggested in any way at all that the application of this specialized helping relationship will act as a miraculous cure for the multitude of pathophysiological conditions with which the nurse is confronted daily. The focus of this process is not so much on the treatment of the illness as it is on supporting the patient through that illness and helping him or her to cope more adaptively with the distress which arises from it.

Fundamental Principles of Client-centred Therapy

Rogers identified a number of fundamental principles which serve to promote growth in individuals, and which are essential to the quality of client–therapist relationships. Central to these is the view that it is the therapeutic relationship itself which exerts the therapeutic effect. In client-centred counselling, the relationship is of the essence, and it is important to note that Rogerian-based strategies are devoid of techniques that involve doing something to or for the client (Gilliland *et al.*, 1984). Rather, it was Rogers' belief that a small and well specified set of personal qualities inherent or developed in the therapist were more important to therapeutic outcome than a set of detailed theories, a collection of specific strategies or techniques, or the possession of long and intensive professional training. For Rogers, the therapist who had the necessary qualities to establish and maintain an effective therapeutic relationship would be more useful as a helper than those in whom such qualities were absent (Bohart & Todd, 1988).

Rogers' conviction that therapeutic outcomes are a function of the qualities of the relationship is still highly relevant today. These qualities may be described within the framework of three major areas: (1) *accurate empathy*, (2) *genuineness or congruence*, and (3) *non-possessive warmth or non-judgemental caring* (Truax & Carkhuff, 1967). Let us consider these in turn.

Accurate Empathy

This refers to the therapist's ability to enter the world of the client, to see things from the client's point of view and to communicate this understanding to the client. It means a careful tracking of the client's verbal and non-verbal communications, based on the sensitive perception of all messages which the client sends out at a given point in time. It also means the capacity of the therapist or helper to communicate this understanding back to the client in a language which both indicates the accuracy of the understanding and a sharing of the essential meaning and feeling of the client's experience. In *On Becoming a Person* (1961) Rogers described accurate empathy in the following way:

> Can I allow myself to enter fully into the world of the patient's feelings and personal meanings and see these as he/she does? Can I step into the private world of the client so completely that I lose all desire to evaluate or judge it? Can I enter it so sensitively that I can move about in it freely, without trampling on meanings which are precious to him? Can I sense it so accurately that I can catch not only the meanings of his experience which are obvious to him, but those meaning which are only implicit, which he sees only dimly or as confusion? (p. 53)

In attempting to clarify this very experimental point of view, Truax & Carkhuff (1967) explain:

> Accurate empathy involves more than just the ability of the therapist to sense the patient's private world as if it were his/her own. It also involves more than just his/her ability to know what the patient means. Accurate empathy involves both the therapist's sensitivity to current feelings and his/her verbal facility to communicate this understanding in a language attuned to the patient's current feelings. (p. 46)

Accurate empathy does not involve the therapist being able to experience precisely the same feelings as the client at precisely the same time; this is neither advisable nor, in most cases, possible. Accurate empathy does, however, involve great sensitivity in listening and in observation so that the therapist is able to pick up and reflect back the breadth of meaning which is contained within the communication. In this way, the client becomes increasingly aware that another person is sufficiently concerned to be listening intently and to want to communicate back the fact that a message, sometimes deeply personal, sometimes obscure, sometimes of a kind which not even the client is fully aware of, has none the less been received and respected by another person. As Rogers (1977) said:

> As the client finds the therapist valuing even the hidden and awful aspects which have been expressed he/she experiences a prizing and liking of him/herself. As the therapist is experienced as being real, the client is able to drop facades, to more openly be experiencing within. (p. 94)

In this sense, the role of accurate empathy within the therapeutic relationship enables the patient to feel trust and comfort in the interaction, and to work towards a willingness to use this relationship in the resolution of problems.

Nurses are in a unique position to listen to their patients, to be sensitive to the messages which are being communicated to them, and to communicate their own understanding of these messages back to their patients in such a way that they indicate a deep personal sharing. Thus, patients who may have believed that they were alone and isolated within the strange and often terrifying environment of the hospital ward or the clinic may come to learn that their fears, concerns and distress are understood and appreciated by one other very important person, the nurse, who also shares that environment. Clearly, as we will see in other chapters of this book, the clinical environment can be a terrifying place for those people who feel they are in a helpless position, and the comfort which they may derive from a knowledge that their distress is understood may mean the difference between rational anxiety and unremitting distress. While this clearly has implications for the patient's sense of wellbeing, it is also likely to make the patient easier to manage, since the patient who knows that his or her fears and concerns are shared and understood is also the patient who is most likely to cooperate with the processes of medical management in which the nurse is a primary participant.

Of course, empathy is not simply something one has by virtue of being a nurse; rather it is an active process or a skill that must be acquired and practised. It is rare for people just to know how another person is experiencing the world. Usually, a person can achieve that knowledge only through a laborious process of listening, adjusting guesses and listening some more. Achieving accurate empathy can take time because it requires clarifying communications between the therapist and the patient. Empathy may mean learning the patient's private language. It requires patience, sensitivity and an understanding of just what empathic listening means. However, within the context of nursing practice, the benefits to be gained from taking the time first to discover the process of empathy and second to listen to one's patients as they express their feelings vastly outweigh any possible inconvenience or expense of time which might be involved in establishing an empathic communication.

Genuineness or Therapist Congruence

For Rogers, genuine people are congruent; that is, they do not have a facade of artificial professionalism that separates them as individuals from their clients. To be congruent nurses must be genuinely themselves: complete, integrated and whole people. This means that their outer actions must be congruent with some facet of their inner thoughts and feelings at any particular point of time. What they say or do must be an accurate reflection of some aspect of what they are currently thinking and feeling. The person (whether it be nurse, counsellor, or therapist in a more formal sense) must be transparent in that there are no facades of emotion or behaviour which may mask honesty and authenticity (Bohart & Todd, 1988; Gilliland *et al.*, 1984). This means that within a therapeutic relationship a nurse's actual experiences are being accurately represented to the patient. In a very real sense therefore, the quality of genuineness, realness or congruence derives from both the attitude and the behaviour or appearance of the therapist, or in this case the nurse (Gilliland *et al.*, 1984).

In *On Becoming a Person* (1961), Rogers refers to genuineness or congruence in the following way:

> How can I be sure that I will be perceived by the other person as trustworthy, as dependable or consistent in some deep sense? How can I be expressive enough as a person that what I am will be communicated unambiguously? I believe that most of my failures to achieve a helping relationship can be traced to unsatisfactory answers to these questions. When I am experiencing an attitude of annoyance towards another person but am unaware of it then my communication contains contradictory messages. My words are giving one message, but I am also in subtle ways communicating the annoyance I feel and this confuses the other person and makes him distrustful, though he too may be unaware of what is causing the difficulty. (pp. 50–51)

In this respect, congruence may be seen to refer to a lack of disparity between the therapist's feelings and behaviours. It means that the therapist must feel comfortable in accepting and admitting to feelings which adherence to convention might ordinarily suppress. The quality of genuineness is associated with openness and self-disclosure (Geldard, 1989).

According to Prochaska (1979), Rogers originally believed that there was no necessity for therapists to speak openly of what they themselves felt to patients. It seemed necessary only that therapists not deceive patients or themselves. Later, however, he came to the conclusion that genuineness in therapists includes their self-expression, and many therapists have begun to follow Rogers' lead of directly expressing some of the emotion and meaning of their own feelings during therapeutic sessions. The justification which they give for this is that such expression allows for a greater perception of congruence of the therapist by the patient. Therapists who speak genuinely of their own feelings are better able to liberate the release and expression of emotional responses and distress in their clients.

It will be seen from this that nurses are once more in a unique position within the medical environment to establish a relationship with their patients which will be truly therapeutic. Their close contact with patients will provide them with opportunities to present themselves as genuine people, in touch with their own feelings and concerns, and therefore by implication able to appreciate and accept the feelings and concerns of those around them. Their capacity to be open and their responses to the medical environment and to their patients will mark them as people who may be trusted and to whom patients may easily talk about feelings of personal distress.

Some people, of course, argue that it is not appropriate for the therapist to disclose all thoughts, feelings or information to the client in a completely open way (Bohart & Todd, 1988). In the hospital setting, concerns about imminent death in terminally ill patients who have not yet come to terms with their illness, or potential incapacity among patients whose injuries are only in the early stages of recovery and treatment, may, if they were communicated in a totally open way to the patient, produce a response which could be either destructive or at odds with the process of maximal recovery and rehabilitation. There will, moreover, be experiences of a purely personal kind unrelated to the work environment or to the needs and concerns of patients which nurses will inevitably bring to their jobs when they switch from private to public roles. We are all subject to difficulties arising with our private lives, and in many respects the intimate details of these difficulties are totally private and personal. A client-centred helping relationship does not demand that every single detail of a therapist's private life (regardless of what role the therapist might be in) is revealed to the patient. It simply encourages the therapist to recognise personal feelings and to be open with patients about feeling these.

It is clear that the nurse who brings a patient's medication and is met by a refusal to take that medication may respond with some anger. Client-centred counselling would encourage the nurse to admit openly to that anger rather than to mask it in expressions of indifference or denial. In this particular instance, the source of the nurse's concern is clear-cut. In other instances, the source may not be so clear-cut. Nurses, as we have said, will bring to their jobs the carry-over of emotional distress and concern about their private lives. While there is no need to reveal the particular aspects of these, the relationship between nurses and patient may well be impaired if nurses are not able to admit to the patient, on questioning perhaps, that they are distracted or concerned or unhappy or angry and that like any normal people, these private concerns may become evident when carrying out their jobs. The essential point to remember is that experiences of concern or emotional reaction are normal and that it is more damaging to a therapeutic relationship to deny or mask these than to admit to their presence and reveal one's self as a real person.

Bohart & Todd (1988) quite explicitly state that when therapists do talk openly about themselves it is frequently in a way which allows growth in their patients. Thus, nurses may use their own personal experiences to demonstrate to the patient that acceptance and expression of concern or distress are normal, natural and acceptable.

Caring or Non-possessive Warmth

The final of the components which Rogers has deemed necessary for the establishment of an appropriate and effective therapeutic relationship is that of caring or non-possessive warmth. This involves the complete acceptance of the patient in a non-judgemental way as the person they are, with all their frailties and weaknesses, and with all their strengths and positive qualities. Having non-possessive warmth does not mean that the therapist must agree with all of the values the patient holds, but simply that the therapist accepts the patient for whatever values are held and does not judge those values according to personal frameworks. This attitude is non-judgemental in the sense that the therapist does not try to impose personal values on to the client or to imply that the therapist's values are in any way superior as a guide to living, or more effective as a means of overcoming personal problems.

Rogers, in *On Becoming a Person* (1961), described the characteristic of non-possessive warmth within the broader context of the term 're-spect', as follows:

> Can I let myself experience positive attitude — attitudes of warmth, caring, liking, interest, respect — towards this other person? It is not easy. I find in myself, and feel that I often see in others, a certain amount of fear of these positive feelings. We are afraid that if we let ourselves freely experience these positive feelings towards another we may be trapped by them. They may lead to demands on us or we may be disappointed in our trust, and these outcomes we fear. So as a reaction we tend to build up distance between ourselves and others — aloofness a 'professional' attitude, an impersonal relationship. (p. 52)

The demonstration of non-possessive warmth enables the patient to feel free and to be open in exploring inner psychological processes without censoring them for fear of criticism. This gives the patient the best opportunity for increased personal awareness and consequent growth (Geldard, 1989). It also acts to increase the patient's own unconditional positive self-regard which is, in Rogers' view of therapeutic change, a crucial element in the resolution of personal difficulties. If the therapist can demonstrate non-possessive warmth for the patient then the patient can begin to perceive more accurately and become more aware of personal experiences that were previously distorted or denied because they threatened a loss of positive regard from significant others (Prochaska, 1979). Thus, by working through this process, the patient may learn to accept experiences, whether positive or negative, which can now be introduced and integrated into the individual's total perception of his- or herself in such a way that actualization or growth is enhanced.

Theoretically it has been suggested that there are actually three inter-related qualities which make up non-possessive warmth. These are (1) that the therapist must actively care for the client, (2) that the therapist's caring must be non-possessive or non-judgemental, that caring should not be contingent on the production of certain 'desired' behaviours in the client, and (3) that the therapist must treat the client with respect as an autonomous and equal partner in the relationship (Bohart & Todd, 1988).

The integration of this trilogy of elements is not surprising in view of the fact that caring is directed towards developing within the patient the capacity for self-evaluation which leads to positive self-regard and growth. It does not mean that the therapist will feel unconditional positive regard or non-possessive warmth at all times for the patient; the therapist who is a normal, open person may feel a whole range of feelings towards the patient, some of which may not be strictly positive. Moreover, the congruent therapist will be able to reveal these negative feelings where they are appropriate. None the less, non-possessive warmth conveys a valuing of the person regardless of the disparity which might exist between the therapist's world and that of the patient.

If there is a difficulty in understanding the role of non-possessive warmth or non-judgemental caring in the nurse–patient relationship, it is that there may be a discordance between the way nurses actually feel about a patient and the way they believe they are expected to respond to that patient. For some, non-possessive caring implies a need not simply to value the individual's right to hold particular attitudes and views but also to share and endorse these values and views. This is not the case, and nurses may give their patients non-possessive warmth simply by recognizing their right to think, believe and act in particular ways.

The most obvious barrier to non-possessive warmth in the nurse–patient relationship is the authoritarian attitude which may derive from professionalism and training. While one would not want to deny the importance of these latter attributes in the nurses' set of skills, nurses must none the less be concerned to ensure that their attitude to their patients is not one of superiority, authoritarianism, disdain and un-concern for their feelings, attitudes and beliefs. They need not share or endorse these, but if they are not respected then the relationship between nurses and their patients may be seriously impaired. As we shall see in later chapters, impairment of this relationship may prove extremely disruptive to the process of care giving.

Evaluating the Effectiveness of Therapeutic Relationships

One of the hallmarks of the Rogerian or client-centred approach to the study of therapeutic relationships is the wealth of empirical evidence which it brings to bear on the effectiveness of such relationships. It is possible to construct scales which allow the measurement of these char-acteristics of a therapeutic relationship. While the scales themselves may be criticized on psychometric grounds (that is, on grounds related to the technical and statistical precision with which they are able to measure the constructs they purport to measure), we have none the less, in client-centred therapy, one of the few areas of the psychological therapies where systematic evaluation has been attempted and has demonstrated the overall usefulness of the area.

Perhaps the best overview of this research is still to be found in the now classic chapter of Truax & Mitchell (1971) entitled 'Research on certain therapist interpersonal skills in relation to process and outcome' which formed part of Bergin & Garfield's monumental work *Handbook of Psychotherapy and Behaviour Change*. Truax & Mitchell summarise the wealth of effectiveness studies in client-centred therapeutic relationships as follows:

> Taken together studies bearing on the systematic evaluation of therapist variables in the study of therapeutic outcome suggest that therapists or counsellors who are accurately empathic, non-possessively warm in attitude, and genuine, are indeed effective. Also, these findings seem to hold with a wide variety of therapists/counsellors, regardless of their training or theoretical orientation, and with a wide variety of patients, including college under achievers, juvenile delinquents, hospitalized schizophrenics, college counsellees, mild to severe outpatient neurotics, and the mixed variety of hospitalized patients. Further, the evidence suggests that these findings hold in a variety of therapeutic contexts and in both individual and group psychotherapy or counselling. (p. 310)

The sum of evidence, both old and new, gives clear-cut support to the assertion that therapists or counsellors, in whatever role they may take on, and this applies to the nursing role as much as any other, will be more effective in their communication and therefore in their general interaction with their patients if they are aware of, and manifest, the characteristics of accurate empathy, congruence and non-possessive warmth.

The area of rehabilitation counselling following acute myocardial infarction provides many examples of the importance of the nurse-counsellor and of the unique relationship which she is able to cultivate and bring to bear on the ultimate recovery and rehabilitation of the coronary patient. This may help illustrate more concretely this important area of nursing practice.

In a wide ranging review of studies examining psychological counselling following myocardial infarction, Doehrman (1977) reported that 10 out of 36 studies involved the nurses as the primary counsellor. A controlled study by Naismith, Robinson, Shaw & MacIntyre (1979) reported that not only were nurses effective counsellors in the context of psychological rehabilitation after myocardial infarction, but that nurses who exhibited the essential therapist variables were most effective in this process. The evidence would, therefore, clearly favour the facilitation of effective counselling skills among nurses since it is clear that in a multitude of areas (and not just those to do with the coronary patient) nurses can effectively contribute to the patient's well-being simply by their capacity to establish a therapeutic relationship with that patient. The issue at hand now is how nurses may acquire the skills necessary to assume this helping relationship with their patients.

Applying Rogers' Principles to Nurse–Patient Relationships

Some take the view that good therapists are born and no amount of formal training, however it is oriented, will compensate for innate difficulties in a person's ability to establish and maintain a therapeutic relationship with another person. This somewhat negative view has been criticized by Truax & Carkhuff (1967) who argue that by a careful understanding of the attributes making up the therapeutic relationship, and by encouraging and practising these attributes, the person in a counselling role, regardless of the context within which the counselling role is exercised, may acquire over time the essential attributes which will make that counselling process most effective. That is, they feel that systematic attention to the necessary ingredients of counselling will help professionals from many disciplines including nursing increase their relationship skills and so their effectiveness as counsellors and helpers. Of course, failure to adopt this view would impart a distinctly pessimistic flavour to the whole notion of helping relationships, since it would assume that only a privileged few would have the capacity to develop and exercise such relationships in a way which would be of benefit to their patients. The evidence is clearly against this view and it is equally clear that relatively simple processes operate in the acquisition and exercise of the therapeutic relationship. What is crucially important is that the helper (whether this be nurse, professional psychotherapist or any other person) is both acquainted with the active ingredients of the therapeutic relationship and is at all times aware of, or at least monitoring for, the presence and expression of these active ingredients in his or her own interaction with patients.

Clearly, it is nurses' responsibility to establish the initial interchange between them and their patients. Patients are demonstrably submissive and dependent within hospital situations, whether they are inpatients or outpatients, and are unlikely, unless they are particularly assertive or aggressive, to begin the process of establishing anything but the most superficial relationships with the nurses who care for them. This responsibility on the nurses' part is an enormous one since the demands on their time, the role expectations which others in their professional world hold for them, their own perceptions of the highly skilled and professionally competent nurse and the essentially goal-directed atmosphere of the hospital environment all mitigate against engaging in relationships with patients which are anything more than task orientated. None the less, the potential advantages of even simple and time-limited helping relationships for the large majority of patients override the inconvenience of such relationships. Over and above the purely concrete issues of convenience, however, nurses may feel reluctant to step beyond their traditional areas of expertise, namely the medical care of the physically ill, for a variety of reasons. They may feel that many others in the hospital environment (psychiatrists, clinical psychologists and social workers) should perform this role and that such trespass into non-traditional areas may result in criticism both by other nurses and by other professionals whose roles are being violated. They may also feel personal discomfort at having to deal with the concerns and sufferings of another person. Such a venture into new territory may both challenge their self-concept as a medical professional with advanced technical training and impose on them interpersonal and emotional demands which they are unwilling or unprepared to assume. Put bluntly, some nurses may feel embarrassment at the prospect of sitting with a patient and sharing fears, concerns and distress in a way which does not directly involve the application of the principles of technological medicine. Others, however, fall into the counselling role naturally and find no difficulty in assuming the helping relationship with all of its implications of listening and sharing. People clearly differ in terms of how easily they can assume such relationships and it is not productive to be critical or judgemental given these individual differences. What is important, however, is the recognition that all nurses have the capacity to acquire the necessary skills to become effective counsellors should they so wish to do.

Early approaches to therapist training took the view that the therapist's work was simply to establish a relationship which allowed clients to get in touch with their most basic feelings. The therapist did this within the context of a helping relationship by demonstrating an attitude of unconditional acceptance of all the feelings which the client expressed and manifested. More current theoretical views on helping relationships suggest, however, that the therapist's work in raising consciousness involves more than just the capacity to feed back to the client a recognition of expressed feeling and a valuing of that feeling. Prochaska (1979) has suggested that the client-centred helper in the context of a helping relationship is a surrogate information processor whose role it is to receive information communicated by the patient, process that information in ways which might be helpful to the patient and then feed back that information to the patient in language attuned to the patient's situation and needs. The nurse in the helping relationship must have the ability to organize emphatically and accurately the information contained within a patient's expressed experience into a concise and complete representation of the patient's own reality, such that the patient not only understands better his or her own experience but comes to realise the value which others give to that experience. The nurse in the helping relationship must act to emphasize the primacy of the individual patient's feelings and concerns, and to empower patients to express fully their feelings at any moment. Such feelings, when they are owned and accepted as coming from within and being worthy of positive regard, will act to facilitate the patient's own self-actualization or growth

(Prochaska, 1979). This will strengthen the patient's capacity to cope with adversity, either in the short term for the duration of the present illness or over the long term. Thus, the nurses' role in initiating and maintaining a very particular and important pattern of communication with their patients can contribute in effective and demonstrated ways to the patients' growth, and by extension, to their capacity to deal with the pain, anxiety and distress of their illness.

Within the framework of both theory and systematic empirical evidence underlying the client-centred or Rogerian approach to the helping relationship, nurses must first acquire at least the rudiments of accurate empathy, congruence and non possessive warmth in order to be successful in using the helping relationship for the good of their patients. This involves some relatively simple exercises which none the less have been carefully developed and evaluated for their contribution to the development of therapeutic skills. We will now consider the simple but important steps which nurses can take in order to equip themselves for the more broadly useful roles of counsellor or helper as opposed to the more limited role of technical operator, important as this may be to the overall and integrated practice of nursing.

The Acquisition of Accurate Empathy

For nurses to have an empathic understanding of their patient's point of view, they must themselves try to view the world from the patient's perspective and communicate these perceptions back to the patient in a language which is attuned to the patient's own understanding and experience. Nurses must become expert listeners, attending not just to the verbal messages but also to the wealth of non-verbal information which the patient conveys. This implies skills of observation within the context of a caring relationship; observation, moreover, which is not coloured by the nurse's own personal frameworks of expectation and acceptability. It also implies interpretation, since the truly empathic nurse will be able to recognize messages contained within the patient's behaviours and expressions of which the patient may only be dimly aware. Rogers emphasized this interpretive process in speaking of the deeper and more sensitive levels of accurate empathy.

Gilliland *et al.* (1984) suggested a series of strategies to facilitate the empathic understanding of a patient's communications. These involve the processes of attending, of verbally communicating empathic understanding and of non-verbally communicating empathic understanding. Each of these processes relies on the nurse's capacity to observe in an open and sensitive way, to receive communications from the patient, to process and understand the information contained within these communications and to feed them back to the patient in a way which promotes understanding and acceptance.

The nurse cannot achieve empathic understanding without attentiveness to the patient: attentiveness that can be sensed by the patient from the beginning. The nurse's attention to the patient involves both an attitude and a skill. To be effective in helping relationships, nurses need to put aside their own reluctance to focus fully on the concerns of the patient, and to do so without sacrificing their own identity and uniqueness. By observing their own behaviour, nurses can perceive whether or not they are attending sufficiently to the patient in a way demanded by the helping relationship. Facial expressions and body posture tell the patient whether the nurse's mind is attuned to what the patient is saying and feeling or whether she is attending at a superficial level only and is directing the major part of her attention to other matters. The physical distance between the patient and the nurse is important to the success of the helping relationship. The nurse who is closely attending will display a physical closeness, certainly with eye contact and perhaps, if the situation requires it, with non-intimate body contact, for example, her hand on the patient's arm. All this can be done without violating the personal space of either the nurse or the patient and any violation of the patient's personal space will almost certainly be communicated back to the nurse by the patient's non-verbal behaviour of physical distancing. Such cues must also always be attended to since they give a clear indication to the patient of the extent to which the nurse is sharing in the diadic (two-way) communication.

Voice qualities such as modulation, tone, pitch, smoothness, diction, enunciation and variation (absence of monotone) also indicate to the patient the degree of attentiveness which the nurse is able to provide. A voice tone indicating disinterest, authoritarian professionalism, uncertainty, a need to hurry away and engage in other activities, dismissiveness, patronization or a belittling of the patient's cares and concerns provides powerful cues to the patient that the nurse is neither attentive nor wishes to be attentive to his or her need to communicate.

Interactions between patients and nurses are almost inevitably coloured by feelings of emotional uncertainty and vulnerability on the part of the patient. These negative feelings can be reduced substantially by nurses who attend to the patient's communications of these feelings and who focus their attention entirely on the patient and on the moment. Nurses who are able to enter the patient's world quickly, skilfully and with care also build trust and eliminate the need for caution among their patients, and are therefore able to establish a helping relationship with greater speed than nurses who are only superficially attentive to their patient's messages.

Attending is, however, only the first step in achieving accurate empathy. Nurses must also develop the capacity to feed back to the patient those communications which they are privileged to receive in the therapeutic interaction. Nurses must relay back to the patient, either verbally or non-verbally, a number of distinct but interrelated messages. First, they must develop the capacity to assure the patient they are listening and understand the essential nature of the message being conveyed. Second, they must communicate to the patient that they respect this message and understand its importance for the patient. Third, they must establish for the patient the assurance that they are there to listen and to help so long as the patient requests this.

The simplest technique for communicating empathy is straight reflection. At this level of empathy, the nurse simply reflects back in similar language and in a similar tone the message which the patient has just communicated. By doing this, the nurse shows the patient, at the very least, that she has understood the surface meaning of that message and that the patient's cares and concerns have been received and registered at a cognitive level. As nurses develop greater skill with simple reflection they may begin to venture into the area of interpretation where they reflect not just the concrete message but the meaning which they believe underlies that message. This of course carries with it the danger that their interpretation will be an incorrect one and that they will communicate back to the patient a misleading or erroneous interpretation. The danger here is not great since patients have enormous tolerance for misinterpretations. Patients will themselves correct misinterpretations which might have been made and are more pleased that someone is attempting to listen than they are displeased that the perhaps subtle nuances of a message have been misconstrued.

Empathy, however, involves not just the verbal communication of received messages but the communication in non-verbal language as well that the essence of the message has been received, interpreted and understood. Changes in body posture, body movement, body position, or facial expression (including smiles, frowns and looks of caring concern), voice quality, eye contact and use of hands can all communicate attention to and understanding of a patient's message.

Of course, not only nurses present their communications both verbally and non-verbally; the patient's own messages may be conveyed as much in non-verbal as in verbal language. Nurses must therefore be attentive both to visual cues and to auditory cues arising from the patient's communications. They must observe as well as listen and take note of what is being conveyed to them by body position and body movement, by the use of posture and the use of hands, and by the tone and qualities of the voice and not just by the straight verbal message. All nurses will be aware that the communication of pain, for example, is seen as much non-verbally as it is in expressions of verbal complaint.

Indeed, in some therapeutic interactions the complete absence of talking and the total reliance on non-verbal message and reflection assumes great importance. The therapeutic silence should not be ignored as a means of communicating caring and concern to a patient. For some patients the burden of pain and suffering or of uncertainty and fear is so great that mere words fail to convey the real meaning of their experience, and under these circumstances the simple presence of the nurse in a helping relationship without the necessity for words can be of untold benefit to the patient's feelings of comfort and well-being.

The importance of accurate empathy for the therapeutic relationship cannot, therefore, be overestimated. Bohart & Todd (1988) summarize this importance in the following ways. First, empathy, along with warmth, creates a sense of trust. Second, it is often therapeutic in itself simply for the patient to feel understood; simply knowing that someone else can understand a patient's feelings may help him or her to feel less alone and more normal. Third, empathy focuses the patients' attentions on what they are experiencing and in effect trains patients to listen to and to try to capture the meanings of that experience. The combined effects of these processes may help patients to cope better and in the long term to achieve a more enjoyable lifestyle.

The Acquisition of Genuineness

For nurses, the acquisition of genuineness involves the dropping of facades which distance them from their patients. The nurse must be aware of any behaviours which attempt to create barriers of authority or aloofness, and establish the communication as a one-way process in which the nurse speaks and the patient receives. In a non-genuine relationship there is a considerable discrepancy between the nurse's verbal expressions and her inner experiencing. This results in a defensive interaction and a distinct lack of congruence between what is experienced and what is being said. For the patient of course, non-verbal messages frequently communicate the nurse's inner experiences and as these messages are at odds with the verbal communications the patient becomes confused and distrusts the nurse's real motives.

Genuineness is achieved if nurses are truly sensitive to their own feelings in the interaction which they have with patients and are able to communicate these feelings in such a way as to ensure the honesty of the relationship. Genuineness demands a great deal of self-awareness and of self-acceptance on the nurses' part. They must constantly scan their behaviour and their verbal messages for double meanings, defensiveness, indications of professional distancing, a wish to maintain artificial roles and a need to be superior to the patient in the relationship. This does not, of course, mean that nurses are unable to exercise the perfectly legitimate professional functions which they must do as a member of a medical team. It does mean that they must be sensitive to and aware of those aspects of their behaviour which might deliberately or otherwise communicate to the patient an unwillingness to engage in a helping, listening relationship. The most fatal error of genuineness is that of mixed messages, and nurses must be particularly aware that their verbal communications are consistent with their non-verbal language since, if they are not, the latter will almost certainly betray the former. The greatest facilitator of genuineness is openness and admission of personal feelings. Patients have remarkable capacities to allow nurses the full expression of their personal feelings, even if these feelings indicate the nurse's own concerns, and genuineness in the nurse–patient relationship can in the large majority of cases be approached without fear of personal judgement.

The Acquisition of Non-possessive Warmth

The essential feature of non-possessive warmth is acceptance. The sensitive communication to the patient that their behaviour, feelings, attitudes and concerns are accepted for what they are does much to establish this important dimension of non-possessive warmth. Acceptance may be communicated verbally, but it may also be communicated by posture or by touch in which the patient is reassured non-verbally that their communications are accepted and respected. Indeed, another important term for non-possessive warmth is respect. If nurses are careful to communicate to their patients that they respect their feelings, attitudes and beliefs, then they are well on the way to achieving non-possessive warmth. In this process nurses must continually scrutinize their own behaviours and communications for signs of judgement. A judgemental attitude to a patient's communication is an effective barrier to non-possessive warmth or caring and can make it difficult to establish an effective therapeutic relationship. Any hint of judgemental dismissiveness inevitably leads to a belief on the patient's part that their attitudes are not respected, that their communications are not valued and therefore that their worth as a person is diminished. Nurses must therefore continue at all times to be sensitive to the nature of their communications and in particular the nature of their responses to messages which the patient gives.

It is felt by some people that non-judgemental warmth or caring is inconsistent with genuineness or congruence since the nurse may have responses to a patient's communication which are fundamentally at odds with the patient's own view. It should be remembered that non-judgemental warmth involves respect but not necessarily sharing or endorsement of the patient's attitudes, beliefs, expressions or behaviours. So nurses are able to disagree or to express a point of view contrary to that expressed by the patient so long as they are careful to communicate back to the patient that they both respect the patient's own point of view and accept their right to hold that particular belief.

Non-possessive warmth, as with genuineness and empathy, involves above all a sensitivity by nurses to themselves as people and as channels of communication back to their patients. Nurses who are aware of their own behaviour, who understand and accept themselves, who are in touch with their feelings and beliefs and who value these as important representations of their persona, who have a clear perception of themselves and are unafraid to present this perception to others will have little difficulty in satisfying all of the requirements which we have discussed for the therapeutic relationship. They will therefore be most effective in using that therapeutic relationship to help their patients achieve physical and emotional comfort, feelings of well-being and perhaps ultimately improve their states of health.

Summary

In this chapter consideration was given to the view that nursing involves a specialized human helping relationship. The nature of helping relationships as defined by psychotherapists was explored. By way of example, it was shown that helping relationships are not only the province of trained mental health practitioners but that nursing also involves a major component of therapeutic care. Carl Rogers' client-centred approach to the helping relationship was explored in detail. Essentially Rogers argued that therapeutic outcomes are a function of the qualities of the helping relationship. In particular, three qualities are highly relevant to positive outcomes in working with patients, namely, accurate empathy, genuineness and non-possessive warmth. Each of these qualities was defined and consideration given to the development of these characteristics in helping relationships. The application of Rogers' principles to nurse–patient relationships was also considered in detail.

The next chapter presents some practical guidelines for counselling patients within the nursing context.

References/Reading List

Bergin, A.E. & Garfield, S.L. (eds) (1971). *Handbook of Psychotherapy and Behavior Change: An Empirical Analysis*. New York: John Wiley & Sons.

Bohart, A.C. & Todd, J. (1988). *Foundations of Clinical and Counselling Psychology*. New York: Harper & Row.

Doehrman, S.R. (1977). Psychosocial aspects of recovery from coronary heart disease: a review. *Social Science and Medicine*, 11, 199–218.

Frank, J.D. (1961). *Persuasion and Healing*. Baltimore: John Hopkins Press.

Fritz, P.A., Russell, C.G., Wilcox, E.M. & Shirk, F.I. (1984). *Interpersonal Communication in Nursing: An Interactionist Approach*.

Norwalk, Connecticut: Appleton-Century-Crofts.

Geldard, D. (1989). *Basic Personal Counselling*. New York: Prentice-Hall.

Gilliland, B.E., James, R.K., Roberts, G.T. & Bowman, J.T. (1984). *Theories and Strategies in Counselling and Psychotherapy*. Englewood Cliffs, New Jersey: Prentice-Hall.

Gordon, D. (1976). *Health, Sickness, and Society*. St Lucia, Queensland: University of Queensland Press.

May, R. (ed.) (1961). *Existential Psychology*. New York: Random House.

Mitchell, K.M., Bozarth, J.D. & Krauft, C.C. (1977). A reappraisal of the therapeutic effectiveness of accurate empathy, nonpossessive warmth, and genuineness. In A.S. Gurman & A.M. Razin (eds), *Effective Psychotherapy: A Handbook of Research*. New York: Pergamon Press.

Naismith, L.D., Robinson, J.F., Shaw, G.B. & MacIntyre, M.M.J. (1979). Psychological rehabilitation after myocardial infarction. *British Medical Journal*, 1, 439–442.

Northouse, P.G. & Northouse, L.L. (1985). *Health Communication: A Handbook for Health Professionals*. Englewood Cliffs, New Jersey: Prentice-Hall.

Perls, F. (1969). *Gestalt Therapy Verbatim*. Lafayette, California: Real People Press.

Prochaska, J.O. (1979). *Systems of Psychotherapy: A Transtheoretical Analysis*. Homewood, Illinois: The Dorsey Press.

Rogers, C.R. (1942). *Counselling and Psychotherapy*. Boston: Houghton Mifflin.

Rogers, C.R. (1957). The necessary and sufficient conditions of therapeutic personality change. *Journal of Consulting Psychology*, 21, 95–105.

Rogers, C.R. (1961). *On Becoming a Person*. Boston: Houghton Mifflin.

Rogers, C.R. (1977). *Carl Rogers on Personal Power: Inner Strength and its Revolutionary Impact*. New York: Delacorte Press.

Stone, G.C., Cohen, F. & Adler, N.E. (1979). *Health Psychology — A Handbook*. San Francisco: Jossey-Bass Publishers.

Sundeen, S.J., Wiscarz Stuart, G., DeSalvo Rankin, E. & Cohen, S.A. (1981). *Nurse–client Interaction: Implementing the Nursing Process*. St Louis: C.V. Mosby Company.

Travelbee, J. (1977). *Interpersonal Aspects of Nursing*. Philadelphia: F.A. Davis Company.

Truax, C.B. & Carkhuff, R. (1967). *Toward Effective Counselling and Psychotherapy: Training and Practice*. Chicago: Aldine.

Truax, C.B. & Mitchell, K.M. (1971). Research on certain interpersonal skills in relation to process and outcome. In A.E. Bergin & S.L. Garfield (eds), *Handbook of Psychotherapy and Behaviour Change: An Empirical Analysis* (pp. 299–344). New York: John Wiley & Sons.

U'Ren, R.C. (1980). *The Practice of Psychotherapy.* New York: Grune & Stratton.
Wexler, D.A. & Rice, L.N. (eds) (1974). *Innovations in Client-centred Therapy.* New York: John Wiley & Sons.

3
Counselling: the Nurse Practitioner's Guide

In Chapter 2 we explored nursing as a helping relationship. This chapter looks at the nature of counselling from a practical point of view. Since nursing is a profession requiring well developed skills in interpersonal interaction, communication and the management of emotional stress, it seems that the need for basic counselling skills is pre-eminent and self-evident.

Nurses are often the first point of contact for patients suffering from emotional distress. Nurses may be required to take on the role of psychiatrist, psychologist or social worker prior to any assistance from professionals trained in these areas. Often nurses are faced with patients feeling suicidal, facing life threatening illnesses or in chronic pain. It is essential, therefore, that nurses become practically familiar with a number of basic counselling skills relevant to dealing with the crises with patients they will commonly encounter.

Basic Qualities

One cannot learn to become an effective counsellor overnight; it takes time, effort and practice. As we indicated in the previous chapter, the psychologist Carl Rogers identified three basic personal qualities which are highly desirable for a counsellor to possess if his or her counselling is to be effective. These qualities, as you will recall, are empathy, congruence and unconditional positive regard. As you may also remember, to be empathic you must feel at one with the patient, to be able to sense communications and to communicate this back to the patient in appropriate ways so as to indicate understanding. To be congruent you must be genuinely yourself in all interactions, a whole and integrated person, not relying on props or facades to present yourself. To display unconditional positive regard you must accept the patient as a person, completely and without any judgements. According to Rogers, and sub-stantiated by a large volume of research evidence, possession of these basic personal qualities, as psychotherapeutic attributes, presaged skilful and effective counselling. Some appear to be born with these qualities, or at least to have developed them at an early age and without formal training or, indeed, the recognition that they carried within them substan-tial power to change behaviour and heal.

Learning to be a Counsellor

Learning to be an effective counsellor is not achieved just through reading books, though there are a large number of excellent texts in this area both on the theory and practice of counselling (see, for example, Gottman & Leiblum, 1974; Brammer, Shostrom & Abrego, 1989; Corsini & Wedding 1989; Prochaska, 1979; U'Ren, 1980; Tschudin, 1982; Nelson-Jones, 1983; Geldard, 1989; Moursund, 1990; Corey, 1986; Gilliland, James & Bowman, 1989). Reading such books as these allows the development of an understanding of what counselling is about, but it is also important to understand how to 'become' a counsellor, and this is best achieved by practical skills training.

Good counselling does require skill and training, and there are tech-niques which must be mastered by those who wish to become profes-sional, full-time counsellors. Broadly speaking, however, training encompasses the complete range of 'helping interactions' which most if not all people engage in, and in fact there are instances where we act as counsellors in our normal day to day activities. When we comfort a friend who is upset, when we listen to an adolescent who is confused about his or her sexuality, or hold the hand of an elderly relative dis-tressed at the loss of an independent lifestyle, we are behaving like a counsellor. And when we take these interactions and others just like them into our occupational settings, just as nurses routinely do, then we are assuming the role of professional counsellors.

Counselling is sometimes spoken of synonymously with psycho-therapy. Frank (1961) defined psychotherapy, in part, as a 'specialized human relationship', and this characteristic is also true for counselling, that is, the interpersonal interaction which forms the necessary basis for the alleviation of psychological distress is common to both. Frank goes on to specify the parameters of this 'relationship', however, by claiming for psychotherapy that one participant (the healer) must have formal training and professional qualifications acceptable to the other participant (the sufferer). It might be argued that here counselling and psychotherapy part company, for the influential research literature on counselling places greater emphasis on the personal qualities of the counsellor (the healer or psychotherapist, in Frank's terminology) than on the formal processes of professional training required to achieve this therapeutic skill. It has also been said that while psychotherapy deals with the treatment of those suffering from relatively severe psychiatric conditions, often using complex techniques of behaviour change, by highly qualified professionals, counselling directs its attention more to the alleviation of individual distress within the 'normal' range of severity and requires far less in the way of professional preparation for its practitioners. Ultimately, of course, the distinction may be more semantic than substantive, since there is little doubt that both rely to a large extent for their effectiveness on the skills of the 'practitioner' in building a working relationship with the 'client' and in using that relationship to promote the client's well-being.

Observation of the activities of professional counsellors reveals a set of interpersonal skills which both identify counselling (as opposed to, say, superficial conversation) and determine its effectiveness in alleviating distress from whatever source it may be seen to arise. These skills (some would call them psychotherapeutic skills) are often closely similar to ordinary but effective skills in interpersonal interaction and communication. Research into the process of counselling suggests that they may be discussed under a number of headings.

Minimal Responsiveness/Matching

Counselling is an extension of what we all do naturally in our relationships with other people when they are hurting (Geldard, 1989, p. 15). Counselling is essentially about *listening*, and listening has been viewed as an active attending process with little or no verbalization (Brammer & Shostrom, 1977, p. 199). One of the most difficult aspects of using the listening technique, it has been suggested, is for the counsellor to keep silent when the patient wants to talk (Brammer & Shostrom, 1977, p. 204). Listening is often thought of as a passive skill; that is, one person does the talking and the other listens. The role of the counsellor, however, is far more than this. The counsellor must also *understand* what the patient is saying and let the patient know that understanding has taken place. The effective counsellor must be responsive in the interaction, in such a way that the patient both experiences being attended to and knows that his or her communications have been received by the counsellor (Moursund, 1990). Being a good listener is an essential skill for effective counselling. By listening with skill, and by repeating with clarity, the counsellor may well make understandable what has been previously confusing to the patient (Bruch, 1981, in Moursund, 1990, p. 14).

There is no need to question a patient about every detail of his or her story. Minimal responses are the best way to assure the patient of the counsellor's full attention. The minimal response is something we automatically do in our conversations when we are predominantly listening rather than talking (Geldard, 1989, p. 21). Minimal responses can, of course, be either verbal or non-verbal; a nod of the head or a 'Uh-hm' are both examples of a minimal response. Quite complex messages may be communicated by equally minimal responses. An 'Ah-ha' combined with a forward body posture may, for example, unmistakably communicate extreme interest to the patient, while a 'Yes' with a backwards reclining posture and folded arms might, with equal certainty, signify a query.

Along with use of the minimal response, it has been found useful to *mirror/match* the patient's posture. If the patient is sitting in a laid-back position with crossed legs, for example, the counsellor may adopt a similar position, so increasing the patient's sense of rapport with the counsellor. Clearly, this may be taken to extremes, with the counsellor being seen either to mimic the patient or spend so much time mirroring/matching that there is an apparent loss of touch with the other modes of communication taking place at the same time. As a general response style, however, the available evidence suggests that mirroring/matching does provide the patient with a sense of closer communication with the counsellor.

Reflections of Feeling and Content

The counsellor's primary role is to listen to the patient, and to attempt to assure the patient that the communicated message has been heard and understood. The counsellor's use of minimal responses together with appropriate matching of non-verbal behavioural (postural) cues is an important first step in establishing links with a patient. After a brief period necessary for the development of the counselling relationship, however, the counsellor must begin to respond more actively to the patient's communications. Simply reflecting the feelings and content of the patient's communications are two straightforward ways in which the counsellor may attempt to draw the patient out and to clarify what is being said in the verbal component of the patient's communications.

If, for example, a tense and distressed patient experiencing symptoms of stress in the occupational situation says to the counsellor 'I haven't stopped working all week. I can't afford time to take lunch breaks and I haven't been able to schedule a game of squash in three weeks. I don't even know what time I'll get home tonight', the counsellor may very simply respond: 'It seems to me like you've had a very busy time at work in the last few weeks'. It may sound, on the face of it, a somewhat trivial and self-evident response, but the counsellor is merely trying to encapsulate what it is that the patient has said, without elaboration, and reflect it back. Reflection of content assists the patient by providing reassurance that the counsellor has heard and understood the message. At least, it tells the patient that the counsellor has been attentively listening, and may (as we will go on to discuss in this chapter) actually work in the direction of bringing the patient to some sense of resolution about a problem or difficulty he or she is currently experiencing.

Reflection of feeling is similar to reflection of content, in that it involves reflecting back information provided by the patient. Reflection of feeling is different from reflection of content, however, as it deals with emotional feelings (often expressed non-verbally as tonal quality of voice, posture, behavioural cues such as gloomy or distressed facial gestures, and the like). Reflection of content is concerned with information and thoughts which make up the explicit, cognitive theme of what the patient is saying (Geldard, 1989, p. 31).

Reflection of feeling has been defined as the attempt by the counsellor to paraphrase in fresh words the essential attitudes (as opposed to the content *per se*) which are being expressed by the patient (Brammer & Shostrom, 1977, p. 182). The important word here is 'fresh'; the counsellor attempts to mirror the patient's thoughts, feelings and attitudes, thereby increasing self-awareness and demonstrating to the patient that what he or she is feeling has been understood by the counsellor.

Paraphrasing, used appropriately, provides highly effective therapeutic responses. Used inappropriately, however, it can easily slow down the process of counselling and irritate the patient. A counsellor who only uses reflections in the counselling interchange may appear to be avoiding the patient's explicit or implicit requests for information, feedback or some other form of assistance; the counsellor may also seem to be hiding behind a professional facade (Moursund, 1990, p. 15), so giving to the patient the impression of only marginal counselling competence. As we saw in the previous chapter, it is important to be genuine in exchanges with patients and this means that even if paraphrasing is inaccurate or not totally 'spot on', it is better for the counsellor to paraphrase what he or she really thinks the patient is saying, even if it is not quite right. More is to be lost in the counselling interchange by being seen as a non-genuine counsellor than as one who is sufficiently genuine to make mistakes and admit to them; showing fallibility may in fact, by reinforcing genuineness, help establish rapport between the counsellor and patient (Moursund, 1990, p. 16).

Feelings are often experienced, as we will see in Chapters 4 and 5, in the form of physiological sensations. A person who is feeling anxious, for example, may have a high heart rate, a red face, and an uneasy stomach. Moreover, feelings are often expressed by patients in a single word such as 'depressed', 'angry', 'sad', or 'happy'. When a counsellor is reflecting back feelings, there is no absolute need to use the word 'feeling'. One problem with using paraphrasing, in fact, is that counsellors may fall into a pattern of using identical words each time. Overusing opening phrases can annoy the patient and worse still can make the patient feel that the counsellor is not really listening at all, but merely responding in a mechanical, even parrot-like fashion (Moursund, 1990, p. 16). It is important, therefore, for the counsellor to be aware of the use of language, continually monitoring personal performance so as to avoid such traps. If a patient has expressed a feeling of sadness, for example, the counsellor might respond by saying 'You're feeling sad', or more simply 'You're sad'. There are always alternatives which may be used so as continually to come across as genuine, attentive and concerned. The important thing is that the patient's feelings are identified and reflected back to him or her by the counsellor at appropriate times. Indeed, reflection of feelings is considered by some (Geldard, 1989, p. 33) to be perhaps the most important of all the counselling skills.

Clearly there are also times when it is appropriate to use both reflection of feeling and reflection of content skills with a patient. For example, when a patient expresses a concern that:

> I don't understand my husband. He never wants to do anything to help me around the house. He won't listen to me. I know I really should confront him and say it isn't fair, but he won't listen. I spend days and days thinking of ways to talk to him about it but there is no point. I know it isn't fair. I should talk to him. But he gets abusive and there is no point.

There is need here both to reflect feeling and content; an appropriate response, encompassing both these skills, might be:

> While you are saying that you believe your husband is not treating you fairly (*content*), you seem also to be saying that you are too afraid to confront him (*feeling*).

There are a number of reasons why reflection appears to be an effective counselling tool. First, reflection helps the patient to feel understood by the counsellor (Brammer & Shostrom, 1977, p. 189). Many patients suffering from psychological disorders or acute and intense emotional reactions to physical illness feel misunderstood most of the time. By reflecting the patient's deepest unverbalized feelings, the counsellor helps the patient realize that these feelings are knowable, both personally and by another person. Second, reflection helps the patient realize that feelings may guide both him or her and the counsellor to an understanding of the causes of disturbed behaviours. Once again, by reflecting the patient's unverbalized feelings, the counsellor may help the patient come to a clarified and simplified understanding of his or her behaviour, and particularly the parts of it that are troubling (Brammer & Shostrom, 1977, p. 191).

Perception Checks

A perception check is similar to paraphrasing, in that it aims to clarify and reinforce what the patient has said. It goes beyond paraphrasing, however, in that it involves the counsellor's inferences about what may be going on for the patient, and requests feedback (from the patient to the counsellor) as to the accuracy or otherwise of the inferences which the counsellor has drawn from the patient's communications (Moursund, 1990, p. 16). For example, a patient may tell the counsellor that 'her mother never listens to her problems'. The counsellor might then respond: 'You are saying that you've talked to your mother over and over again about your problems but she never seems to listen. This makes you feel very angry. Is that the case?'. This response involves *paraphrasing* together with an *inference*. It is essential that the accuracy of the inference is determined before proceeding with the counselling interchange. Sometimes, a perception check may result in greater awareness on the part of the patient; in the instance outlined above, the inference regarding anger may not have consciously occurred to the patient, who now gains further insight into her feelings and difficulties. On other occasions, the inference made by the counsellor will be wholly inaccurate, and the use of a perception check allows the counsellor to establish this accuracy before continuing with perhaps an erroneous view of the patient's feelings and difficulties. Whatever the outcome of the perception check, the counsellor must accept the patient's response to the inferences that have been made, and proceed from there with the counselling interchange.

Summarizing

Summarizing what the patient has said can also allow for checks of the counsellor's understanding of what is happening in an interaction, and may possibly increase the patient's self-awareness of his or her problem. It can help in those times when the interaction between a counsellor and patient has, for whatever reason, become stuck. It allows for a stocktake of ideas by the counsellor, and encourages the counsellor to focus more on those areas in the counselling relationship requiring further work (Moursund, 1990, p. 17). Whatever the reason, summarizing always involves the counsellor gathering together the main issues which have been discussed with the patient to that point, and using this summary of issues to review, confirm or correct the points which have been considered, the inferences drawn and the directions taken in counselling.

Questioning

The use of questions in counselling can be also helpful at times, though it is believed that their usefulness is limited and that they should only be employed in a very specific manner in counselling. For the most part, if the counsellor is attentive to the patient's communications, and reflects back both content and feelings in a sensitive, exploratory manner, there is little need for explicit questioning. Indeed, many experienced counsel-lors carefully avoid asking direct questions of the patient because of the way in which questioning can interrupt or distort the flow of a counsel-ling interaction or, indeed, impede a counselling relationship built up as much on personal interaction as explicit verbal content (Moursund, 1990, p. 22). Questioning may, however, be necessary where there is a need to gather a large amount of information as accurately and succinctly as possible, and in a short period of time.

Questions directed to this end tend to be of two types, *open ended* and *closed ended*. Both types of question can be useful in the counselling process, and particularly that part of it requiring the direct collection of information, if used appropriately.

Closed-ended questions are used if a specific piece of information must be collected. For example, questions like 'How old are you now?' or 'Are you feeling sad today?' will tend to lead to a specific and hope-fully factual disclosure. There are times when a counsellor simply needs to know specific biographical information (how many children, marital status and the like) and closed-ended questions are entirely appropriate in those instances. The trouble with closed-ended questions is that they limit the sort of answer the patient can give. A patient, in response to a question 'How many children do you have?', may correctly infer from the nature of the question and from its tone that only the facts are being sought by the questioner, and reply simply 'five'. She does not feel permitted by the nature of the question to add that they are all under the age of six, that she is having considerable trouble caring for them, and that she harbours negative feelings towards them for this reason. In most instances, the aim of counselling is to open up rather than close off dialogue, and consequently closed-ended questions should be used when only the facts are needed. The patient referred to above may have provided a completely different response to a question such as 'Would you like to tell me something about your present family situation?'.

Open-ended questions allow the patient considerably more freedom than closed-ended ones to provide information which they believe to be important. The counsellor may adopt a number of simple questioning strategies to allow the patient that freedom. Instead of specifying the subject of the enquiry by asking, for example, 'Are you sad?', the counsellor may ask the patient 'How are you feeling today?'; instead of 'Are you married, single, divorced, widowed or in a *de facto* relation-ship?', the counsellor may simply ask, 'Can you tell me a little bit about your home situation?'. This allows the patient not only to give the required biographical information but also, should he or she feel so moved, to share with the questioner something of the quality of that situation and of the difficulties (or indeed, the joys) which might accom-pany it.

Open-ended questions, then, are far more useful in counselling than closed-ended questions, because they allow the patient to explore areas of concern without feeling constrained by the nature of the question to provide factual information and nothing else. By being given the freedom and the encouragement to open up in this way, the patient is able to disclose more and to share more with the counsellor than is ever likely if the counsellor used only closed-ended questions.

As we have indicated above, questions, when used with careful phrasing and discretion, can be helpful in the counselling situation. There are, however, a number of problems with the extensive use of questions in counselling. As we stated earlier, many experienced counsellors attempt to avoid using questions at all, if possible. They do so because direct questions may lead to mistakes, both in the process of counselling and in the information which may be derived. The common mistakes which naive counsellors appear to make in using questioning techniques in counselling have been identified by research in the area, and three are discussed below.

First, the counsellor takes exclusive control of the interaction, and expectations regarding patterns of communication in the counselling relationship develop which are hard to change. The counsellor alone therefore comes to dictate the topics to be considered and the direction of the interaction. The effect of this is twofold: the counsellor will almost certainly fail to perceive or appreciate much of what is important to the patient, and the patient in turn may never have the opportunity to take personal responsibility for his or her own behaviour.

Second, the counsellor attempts to coerce the patient into answering questions according to (the counsellor's) preconceived expectations of responses. For example, the counsellor may use a questioning session to push the patient down a particular path, by phrasing questions in terms such as, 'What you really meant to say there was . . .', or 'Don't you really mean that . . .'. Alternatively, and perhaps more simply, the counsellor may continually repeat the same question until the patient gives the answer that the counsellor wants to hear. This does not imply a conscious attempt by the counsellor to falsify information pertinent to a patient, but, more subtly, a need by the counsellor to confirm or reinforce particular attitudes or points of view. Most counsellors have preconceptions about the problems which patients present to them. Persistent questioning may allow those preconceptions to prevail.

Third, the counsellor attempts to interpret for the patient. Questions like 'Do you still hold a grudge against your father for the way he treated you?', or 'Do you want the same things from your relationships now that you wanted as a child?' are examples of interpretative questions. Unlike coercion, the counsellor has a reasonable hypothesis about where the patient is, but phrases questions so as to limit information which might bear on other, equally reasonable hypotheses in an attempt to get confirmation of the favoured hypothesis.

Since the temptation to take control, coerce and interpret may be very strong for some counsellors, it is important for all those in counselling situations to guard against the use of questions directed to these ends. Moursund (1990, pp. 23–24) has argued that there are a number of guidelines which careful counsellors should follow when using questions during counselling sessions with patients. The counsellor should:

1. only ask questions when really necessary — the patient will feel more in control if allowed to build his or her structure rather than having to follow someone else's;
2. make sure the patient knows that the question arises from the counsellor's own confusion when asking questions for clarification, to avoid reinforcing a belief that it arises from something the patient has done wrong;
3. avoid closed-ended questions wherever possible — these shift responsibility for information reporting away from the patient and onto the counsellor which, as we have seen, is to be avoided;
4. use open-ended questions to fill in gaps in the patient's story;
5. never insist that a patient answer set or posed questions if there is reluctance to do so;
6. always use questions which help the patient to take responsibility for decisions and find personal solutions to problems.

Confronting the Patient

There are times, however, typically after attempts to increase a patient's self-awareness have failed, when it is appropriate to use confrontation techniques. In counselling, confrontation is used to bring into the patient's awareness, in a sensitive and acceptable way, information which may be personally unpalatable and which is either being avoided by the patient or is just not being noticed (Geldard, 1989, p. 65), presumably, in the counsellor's view, to the patient's detriment. Accordingly, Geldard (1989, p. 67) has identified situations in the counselling process when confrontation is considered to be appropriate. These are when:

1. the patient appears to be avoiding an issue which is apparently troubling;
2. the patient is failing to appreciate self-destructive or self-defeating behaviour;
3. the patient is failing to appreciate the possibly serious consequences of personal behaviour;
4. the patient is not in touch with reality;
5. the patient is making multiple statements, some of which are contradictory to one another;
6. the patient is excessively and inappropriately focused on the past or the future and is unable to focus on the present (including the present problems);

7. the patient's accounts or explanations of difficulties are going around in circles; and
8. the patient's verbal and non-verbal behaviours conflict, or at least do not match each other.

It is important to note that the counsellor necessarily makes judgements of a patient's words, thoughts and behaviours in arriving at a conclusion that each or any of these situations exists. There may be no absolute objectivity in the evaluation of situations foreshadowing confrontation; the counsellor must assimilate and assess the total set of circumstances, including not only the patient's words, thoughts and behaviours, but also the context in which these appear. Confrontation is a positive technique which challenges the patient rationally to reassess his or her own words, thoughts and behaviours, but it may also be experienced as personally threatening by a patient unsure of the level of trust engendered in the relationship with the counsellor. Only after a sensitive and careful evaluation of the complete situation, therefore, should the counsellor choose to confront the patient. In such instances, the counsellor may confront the patient by (Geldard, 1989, p. 67):

1. reflecting what the patient has said, and challenging the patient rationally to reconsider the content of the message;
2. stating what the counsellor is personally feeling in the relationship, so inviting the patient to share the counsellor's concern; and/or
3. stating the counsellor's observations of the patient's words, thoughts and behaviours in the counselling relationship, but offering no interpretation.

The aim of confrontation is not to attack the patient but to convey the message that the counsellor understands and cares about the problem. An example might help to clarify the practice of confrontation in the process of counselling. Consider the following: A patient has been been suffering from depression for some time, and constantly and excessively refers during counselling to the breakdown of a friendship which occurred a decade or more ago. While this was discussed at length, and the patient had agreed with the counsellor that it was time to move on and focus on the here and now, he continues at each counselling session to return to the events of years past, unable to accept resolution of these and move on to fresh and more fruitful areas of discussion.

The counsellor, in turn, feels confused and frustrated because no headway has been made in dealing with the patient's depression, and the patient continues to suffer. The counsellor may then feel the need to confront in order to bring this situation to a conclusion:

> I'm confused. While you seem to be saying that you want to deal with your current difficulties, you continue to talk about a past event. Perhaps we should agree that you can't change what is in the past but you can do

something about the present. If we take this as 'said', I think we can make more progress with counselling than if we are working at different levels.

This sort of confrontation is not at all attacking, but simply and honestly seeks to clarify, establish ground rules and enhance the effectiveness and efficiency of the counselling process. As the example shows, confrontation of this kind would be useful where patients are preoccupied with historical events (as so many people in distress seem to be) at a time when sorting out present difficulties would be more appropriate and more likely to restore psychological equilibrium and alleviate psychological distress.

Specific Counselling Skills

So far, we have looked at some general counselling skills (reflection, summarizing, questioning, confrontation and so on) which are likely to prove useful in nursing practice. There are a number of patient groups, however, which nurses are more likely to encounter than others in the course of their professional activities. These are angry patients, grieving patients, suicidal patient and patients in severe or chronic pain. Because of their frequency in nursing practice, they are worthy of special attention, and nurses should have an understanding of ways to work with such patients.

Angry Patients

Nurses frequently have to deal with angry patients. The nature of anger is more fully discussed in Chapter 5 on the emotions; however, simple human experience will tell nurses that patients who are experiencing or expressing substantial levels of anger are, at the very best, difficult to communicate with. There are also times in nursing practice when encountering another person's anger can be very frightening for nurses, even if they are not the recipients of the emotion. Some techniques for dealing with experienced or expressed anger are therefore likely to be of real practical use for nurses.

The identification of anger in the clinical situation, as we shall point out in Chapter 5, is relatively clear-cut. Patients will become withdrawn and uncooperative, communicating infrequently and poorly with those caring for them, and sometimes having outbursts of verbally or physically aggressive behaviour. Whether the anger is controlled or evident as aggressive behaviour, two initial and simple ways are available to assist with the control of anger. The first is to encourage the patient to express openly feelings of anger in the context of a supportive and caring environment, seeking to verbalize feelings realistically but without need for aggression. Of course, there are times when expression of angry feelings needs to reflect the extremity of the difficulties being experienced. None the less, controlled expression of anger may act as a safety valve to protect the patient from the more damaging effects which suppression of that emotional state may cause (see Chapter 5). Secondly, the nurse may elect to teach the patient to relax, so providing the patient with the means of self-control and of alleviation of both psychological and physical distress which accompanies the experience of anger (we will discuss the techniques of relaxation below). In the longer term, it may also be possible to help the patient to examine mechanisms not just for releasing but also for overcoming anger (Geldard, 1989, p. 121), though this is a psychotherapeutic exercise with a specialized technology requiring considerable skill in counselling (Novaco, 1975).

The simple, verbal release of anger can be effectively achieved through the reflective techniques described above in this chapter. The counsellor quite simply reflects back the anger perceived in the patient's communications, so as to make the patient aware that this anger has been understood and may be expressed without disapproval. In situations of extreme anger, however, it may be better to use the method developed from *gestalt therapy*. Geldard (1989, pp. 121–122) has suggested the following brief procedure for use in this situation:

1. First, just ask the patient to identify the source of their anger ('Who or what are you angry with?').
2. Then, place an empty chair about a metre away from, but facing, the patient.
3. Say to the patient, 'Imagine that the person (or object) who is the target of your anger is sitting in the empty chair'.
4. Continue by asking the patient to 'talk to the imaginary person (or object) sitting in the empty chair about your angry feelings'.
5. If necessary, help the patient to express anger fully and openly by 'coaching' — this can be achieved by standing alongside the patient and repeating, in more forceful tones than the patient's initial attempts, the comments made by the patient to the imaginary person (or object) in the empty chair, until the patient is able to verbalize completely that anger with appropriate vehemence.

This is just one example of an alternative method to strategies emphasizing the simple reflection of feelings, to encourage the angry patient to externalize and express their unpleasant feelings. It does so constructively, without the need for extreme aggression, and in a manner which the patient may find novel and therefore attractive. So-called 'empty chair' techniques have a wide use in counselling where there is a need for the patient to focus on a particular emotional state brought about in response to a specific person, object or situation. The capacity to focus emotion onto a symbolic representation of the offending person or object makes the expression of that emotion more real than if it were simply reflected back, in an abstract sense, by the counsellor. The effectiveness of this set of techniques is well demonstrated in the counselling literature.

Progressive Muscle Relaxation

As we stated earlier, however, another strategy which counsellors can use to assist angry patients is that of systematic *muscle relaxation therapy*. Muscle relaxation therapy, sometimes called *progressive relaxation training*, is a well established technique in clinical and counselling psychology used to produce deep muscle relaxation and, as a consequence, an overall reduction in levels of physiological arousal underlying states of severe psychological distress. The physiological and psychological bases for this are discussed in the following chapter on stress. Briefly, muscle relaxation therapy uses a set of structured exercises involving both contraction and relaxation of specific muscle groups, sometimes accompanied by appropriately relaxing mental imagery, to train individuals to achieve states of relaxation quickly, easily and whenever the situation demands. Thus, angry patients, for example (or anxious or depressed patients), can, on recognizing the presence of anger or other emotional distress, use muscle relaxation strategies to counteract the unpleasant emotional state and replace it with the more comfortable and adaptive state of relaxation. The theoretical basis for this is called *reciprocal inhibition*, meaning simply that the imposition of relaxation onto a situation characterized by intense unpleasant emotion acts to inhibit the unpleasant emotion, replacing it instead with a state of relaxation. Once more, there is abundant evidence in the psychological literature on the operation and merits of this technique in the treatment of emotional distress.

While there are many different approaches to systematic or progressive relaxation training, some almost entirely based on muscle contraction/relaxation exercises and others focusing as well on mental imagery strategies, all can be used to alleviate emotional distress. The following procedure represents a typical, if very detailed and comprehensive method.

1. Enquire into the patient's problems, precipitating difficulties and past experiences with counselling or other psychotherapy (as a means of collecting information used to guide counselling and assist in the selection of the appropriate relaxation strategy. As we will discuss shortly, not all patients respond to relaxation exercises in the same manner, and individual preferences must be taken into account in the choice, for example, of active (muscle contraction/relaxation) or passive (imagery based) strategies.)

2. Introduce the idea and purpose of progressive muscle relaxation so that the patient knows what he or she might expect of the exercises.

3. Demonstrate and begin the practice of relaxation, focusing on detailed, individual muscle groups.

4. Establish the routine of practice at home and arrange additional clinic sessions if required.
5. Once basic relaxation skills are established, work towards the shortening of the procedure to fewer muscle groups (this usually requires two further sessions plus some regular home practice).
6. Continue to shorten further the procedure to just a few muscle groups (this usually requires two more sessions plus further regular home practice).
7. Finally, shorten the procedure even further by omitting the muscle contraction component of the exercises and achieving relaxation by mental command alone.

General Guidelines
Patients considered for muscle relaxation therapy are told that simply knowing about progressive relaxation procedures will not induce relaxation. It must be practised regularly and diligently until it can be induced effortlessly and quickly whenever it is required. Patients are advised that they must set aside two periods of 20 to 30 minutes each day for basic practice of the exercises. As relaxation skills become established, they are extended beyond the clinic, the hospital ward or the home into everyday settings where psychological distress normally occurs. Patients are also advised that they should only practice their initial attempts at muscle relaxation when (1) they are in a safe, comfortable environment where they are unlikely to feel threatened or to be disturbed, (2) they are not under pressure to finish the exercises and meet other deadlines, and (3) they are sufficiently awake and attentive to the procedure that they are unlikely to fall asleep during the exercises. Relaxation exercises should be carried out in a completely comfortable bodily position, typically on a couch or bed, such that all areas of the body are supported and there is no need for muscle tension to maintain posture. It is, moreover, recommended that a note pad and pencil be kept handy so that after each session some notes can be made of problems arising during the relaxation exercises, or of questions which might need to be discussed with the counsellor.

The Exercises
Each muscle group is moderately contracted (tensed), but not uncomfortably so, for 5 to 7 seconds, then relaxed for around 30 seconds. If necessary, the exercise for any single muscle group is repeated once or twice before moving on to the next muscle group. Patients are told that they should not tense a muscle so hard that physical discomfort follows — moderate tension is quite effective for the exercise. Patients are also told not to force relaxation, but to let it happen. When relaxing, they are instructed to focus their attention on relaxing more and more with each breath they take — concentration on breathing becomes an integral part of muscle relaxation. Patients are asked to say silently to themselves the

word 'relax' each time they exhale, thus learning to associate a mental stimulus, the silent repetition of the word relax, with the physiological response of relaxation. In this way, over time, the association allows the physiological response of relaxation to occur simply as a consequence of the silent utterance of the word relax.

When tensing, patients are instructed to concentrate on their awareness of the feelings of tension in the muscles, and when relaxing, to concentrate on how much the muscles are becoming more and more relaxed as the exercises progress. Awareness, too, is an integral and important part of the process of muscle relaxation training, both as a direct cue to the patient that a muscle group requires relaxation, and as a form of monitoring that relaxation is actually taking place in response to the practice of the exercises.

In the very beginning of a muscle relaxation program, as we have said, the patient must learn to relax specifically a relatively large number of individual muscle groups. A typical set of exercises might follow the pattern set out below, and the counsellor takes the patient through the complete set of exercises, assessing progress, checking for difficulties and reassuring the patient at all times on progress. The program might attend, in order, to the following:

1. *the muscles of the dominant hand and forearm*, asking the patient to make a tight fist, hold the tension for 5 to 7 seconds, feel (become aware of) the tightness in the hand and forearm and then relax this muscle group for 30 seconds before repeating the exercise or going on to the next one;

2. *the biceps muscles of the dominant side*, instructing the patient to tense these by pushing the elbow down and drawing it in towards body (but leaving the hand and forearm relaxed), hold the tension for 5 to 7 seconds and then relax this muscle group for 30 seconds before repeating or moving on;

3. *the muscles of the non-dominant hand and forearm*, duplicating the exercise set out in (1) above, for this side of the body;

4. *the non-dominant biceps muscles*, duplicating the exercise set out in (2) above for this side of the body;

5. *the muscles of the upper face*, where the patient is asked either (whichever seems the best way for the patient) (a) to raise the eyebrows as high as possible, hold for 5 to 7 seconds, feel the tension and then relax for 30 seconds, or (b) draw eyebrows down and frown, hold for 5 to 7 seconds, feel the tension and then relax this muscle group for 30 seconds;

6. *the muscles of the middle face*, for which the patient is instructed to squint the eyes tightly and at the same time wrinkle the nose, holding the tension for 5 to 7 seconds, becoming aware of the tension and then relaxing this muscle group for 30 seconds;

7. *the muscles of the lower face*, for which it is suggested that the patient should clench the teeth firmly together and pull corners of

the mouth back, and then hold for 5 to 7 seconds, feeling the tension before relaxing this muscle group for 30 seconds;

8. *the neck muscles*, where the patient is told to pull the chin down toward the chest but at the same time try to prevent it from touching the chest (the muscles at the front of the neck should be 'pushing' against those at the back), then holding for 5 to 7 seconds, becoming aware of the tension and finally relaxing this muscle group for 30 seconds;

9. *the muscles of the shoulders* for which the patient should draw the shoulders up as if on strings, then hold for 5 to 7 seconds, feel the tension and relax this muscle group for 30 seconds;

10. *the muscles of the chest, shoulders and upper back*, which may be relaxed by taking a deep breath, holding it for 5 to 7 seconds while at the same time pulling the shoulder blades together, becoming aware of the tension and then relaxing this muscle group for 30 seconds;

11. *the stomach muscles*, where the patient is instructed to make the stomach hard and tight (as if anticipating a direct blow), then holding for 5 to 7 seconds, feeling the tension and relaxing this muscle group for 30 seconds;

12. *the muscles of the right upper leg*, for which the patient is told to push the upper large muscle of the upper leg downwards and in opposition to the smaller muscles underneath, and having done this, to hold the tension for 5 to 7 seconds, become aware of the tension and then relax this muscle group for 30 seconds;

13. *the muscles of the right calf or lower leg*, where the patient should tense these muscles by pulling the toes upward and toward the head, holding the tension for 5 to 7 seconds, feeling the tension and then relaxing this muscle group for 30 seconds;

14. *the muscles of the right foot*, instructing the patient to curl the toes down towards the surface of the foot (but not too hard so as to avoid cramping of the foot), hold the tension for 5 to 7 seconds, feel the tension and then relax the foot for 30 seconds;

15. *the muscles of the left upper leg*, by repeating the exercise set out in (12) above for this side of the body;

16. *the muscles of the left calf or lower leg*, by repeating the exercises set out in (13) above for this side of the body;

17. *the muscles of the left foot*, by repeating the exercises set out in (14) above for this side of the body.

Used correctly, relaxation strategies have considerable potential in counselling and psychotherapy. They allow the counsellor to rapidly intervene with patients suffering severe emotional distress of whatever kind, and to achieve benefits which are immediately apparent both to the counsellor and the patient. The counsellor must, as we have already emphasized, lead the patient through these exercises. Each exercise may be repeated once, or twice if either the patient or the counsellor feel it is needed. The pace of the exercises may be tailored to the patient's unique requirements, and if the counsellor is an experienced relaxation therapist, the exercises themselves may be varied to suit individual preferences. The set of exercises outlined above is by no means the only way to achieve progressive muscle relaxation through training programs. These exercises rely largely on muscle contraction/relaxation procedures first set out in the 1930s by the physiologist Jacobson. Some relaxation therapists, by contrast, focus more on imagery-based techniques, asking the patient to relax by imagining, as vividly as possible, a scene or situation which he or she personally finds relaxing. The merits of this arise from the view that some patients find the process of active muscle contraction unpleasant or even painful, and feel more in control when allowed to achieve relaxation just by imagination. The evidence, however, suggests that only a few patients, largely those not particularly tense or distressed, benefit from this approach. Patients suffering more severe degrees of distress are usually not able to come close to relaxation by imagination alone, and require the more active techniques, at least in the first instance, in order to achieve relaxation. Thus, active relaxation based on contraction/relaxation procedures, as outlined above, appears to be the method of choice to begin with.

There are some patients, however, for whom this technique is legitimately aversive. Patients with muscle or bone weakness or other orthopaedic difficulties, for example, will find even moderate muscle contraction relatively unpleasant and even painful. They may also fear the potential consequences, reasonable or not, of placing muscle strain or pressure on parts of their bodies they perceive to be vulnerable. Occasionally, this only applies to particular components of the relaxation exercise program. If it poses any problem at all, the patient should be evaluated medically and an experienced relaxation therapist, usually a clinical psychologist, should be consulted regarding alternative relaxation procedures. There is some evidence that the muscle contraction/relaxation exercises outlined above, in that they involve *isometric procedures* (those where one muscle group acts in opposition to another to achieve contraction), may also tax a vulnerable cardiovascular system, increasing blood pressure and perhaps precipitating episodes of anginal chest pain in cardiac patients. Once more, where there is doubt, a medical opinion should be sought prior to employing such relaxation procedures. Three rules should always be remembered in this regard. First, where there is doubt about physiological or anatomical vulnerability to relaxation procedures, check it out with the patient's physician. Second, if any relaxation exercise causes pain or discomfort to the patient, discontinue that exercise immediately and caution the patient against attempting the exercise alone. Finally, there are always alternative exercises using less active procedures, and a clinical psychologist can advise on their use.

As you can see, the progressive relaxation training technique requires time, training and patience. It has been considered under the heading of 'Angry Patients' because it is of demonstrated use in this situation. It is also of considerable use, as we have said, in the management and counselling of a large range of other patients suffering from a diversity of forms of emotional distress. Anxious patients, depressed patients, patients failing to cope with the stress of illness may all find benefit from relaxation training programs, as will women preparing for childbirth, young patients in rehabilitation after a serious illness or injury, or middle-aged men recovering from heart attacks. Indeed, nurses themselves will benefit from learning relaxation techniques when dealing, for example, with the potential effects of burnout in their stress-prone occupation, and we will be discussing this further in Chapter 9.

Strategies for dealing with a patient's future anger are more complicated and would generally be beyond the scope of the activities or counselling skills required of most nurses engaged in routine clinical practice. Various methods, including role-playing and the use of 'thought stopping' techniques, have been suggested as effective strategies to control anger (Geldard, 1989, pp. 126–131), and the interested reader might wish to pursue these. Nurses are certainly likely to encounter many patients who are feeling angry, or either overtly or covertly expressing anger, and there will be times when the intensity of this anger will be overwhelming for the patient. There will also be times when it will appear frightening for the nurses physically caring for the patient. In many instances, the course and presentation of the anger will be complex, and the cause not always obvious, so that simple techniques such as those we have just discussed will be insufficient to control the emotion. In such instances, it is appropriate immediately to refer the case to a qualified counselling practitioner such as a clinical psychologist whose role it is to spend time with the patient in order to explore and modify this behaviour.

Grieving Patients

The care of the physically ill frequently brings the carer into contact with real or threatened loss (see Chapter 5 for a more complete account), the expected response to which is depression or grief. Nurses are often involved in helping patients handle some sort of loss and the grief this carries with it. The loss may relate to the death of another person, personal life threat, the breakdown of a relationship, the surgical removal of a bodily organ, the real or threatened loss of physical integrity or capacity, and the corresponding loss of self-esteem; in the practice of nursing, the possibilities for encountering situations of loss are enormous. Whatever the cause, the process of grieving is an extremely painful one for those experiencing it, and a sensitive and difficult one for those in the caring role.

When counselling someone who is grieving, it is important to re-assure him or her that he or she is not alone and that others have and will continue to grieve. Reflection of feeling techniques should be used to encourage the patient to explore his or her feelings fully and openly.

The process of grieving typically follows a number of stages occurring in a fixed sequence, and Geldard (1989, pp. 133–136) has described them as:

1. shock — the person appears to be numb, behaviourally and cognitively immobilized, and incapable of any action;
2. denial — the person cannot believe (or refuses to believe) that what is happening is really true, choosing instead to cling to the delusion that it is a mistake, a myth, a dream or a cruel trick;
3. emotional, psychological and physical symptoms — the person may go on to experience symptoms of emotional despair, depression and feelings of hopelessness and worthlessness, as well as somatic symptoms such as loss of appetite, insomnia and generally impaired physical health;
4. guilt — the person may then blame themselves for what has happened, believing the loss to be a direct consequence of (perhaps even punishment for) their own behaviours or past misdeeds;
5. anger — the person, having resolved or rationalized guilt, may then blame others for what has happened, including members of the hospital staff (perhaps even you), or in the case of suicidal death, the very person whose loss they are grieving for;
6. idealization — the person may, in the process of grieving, put aside all memories of the faults and inadequacies of their lost object (whether person, bodily part, role or self-concept), focusing only on idealized, positive aspects of that which has been lost;
7. realism — the person begins, as the grieving process continues, to accept the loss as a painful but permanent reality; and
8. acceptance, readjustment and personal growth — the person finally and actively seeks new experiences, attempting in the process to move ahead of grief and into a new existence of which the lost object is no longer a tangible part.

Being aware of the stages of grief is the first step in the counselling or management of the grieving patient. The most immediate implication of this is that grieving is a process with a very definite time course, and is for the most part self-resolving. Some people, however, whatever their focus of grieving, may fail to negotiate one or other of the stages, becoming fixated on the essentially maladaptive behaviours characteristic of that phase. The counsellor's role, having identified the problem phase, is to lead the patient empathically towards resolution, using reflection and, if necessary, confrontation so that the patient is able to complete the process and achieve acceptance. Grief counselling is a complex area, with a set of techniques deriving largely from crisis intervention therapy (Gilliland & James, 1988). These techniques rely on a careful identification of the level of grief and its precipitant (the loss), the use of basic counselling skills to create a relationship in which the patient is able to share the grief and work through to its resolution, and the establishment of support networks outside of the counselling relationship to allow for more broadly based contact in times of most distress. Gilliland & James (1988) emphasize the great range of circumstances in which loss may precipitate grief, and from this it is clear that grief is not restricted simply to bereavement or situations of a similarly traumatic magnitude. It is also clear that in many instances, since loss is so closely bound to illness, the nurse will often be the first contact point in a possibly long chain of caregivers necessary for the patient's full recovery. None the less, as with an angry patient, a grieving patient may overtax the counselling skills of the busy, clinical nurse, and may certainly place time demands upon her which are not easy to meet. In this instance, referral of the difficult patient to a skilled counsellor experienced in grief counselling may well be the most important step the nurse can take.

Suicidal Patients

In hospital settings, it is unfortunately all too common for people to be admitted to a casualty unit as a consequence of failed suicide attempts. The issue of the rights and wrongs of attempting to take one's own life is a vexed question, and we will not deal with it here. Whatever your personal view, however, the reality is that suicidal patients are very often intent on killing themselves eventually (Geldard, 1989, p. 137), and their hurt must be taken seriously. You may hope that as practising nurses you will not be called upon to manage a suicidal patient, but chances are that you will; it comes as part of the professional responsibility of nursing.

There are many reasons why people may decide to take their own lives. Geldard (1989, p. 138) has divided suicidal people into three categories, these being:

1. the chronically ill, those in chronic pain, the seriously disabled, those in extreme poverty — in all instances, there appears little hope for improvement;
2. those who have suffered a severe emotional trauma and are in a state of profound depression;
3. those who use suicidal talk or behaviour as a last resort in an effort to get others to hear or respond to their emotional hurt — in some instances, there may be an element of manipulation and an ambivalence towards dying.

Dealing with a patient who has attempted suicide or who you believe may attempt suicide is extremely frightening for many counsellors. Indeed, of all persons with whom nurses deal, a suicidal patient is perhaps the most demanding and the most frightening (Moursund, 1990, p. 112). A suicidal patient make evoke pity in the counsellor, but may equally bring on the counsellor's anger in response to the perceived 'stupidity' of the behaviour. Suicide is an act well able to produce highly judgemental attitudes in otherwise rational and dispassionate health professionals. The recurrent suicide attempter can certainly provoke anger among nurses who may, only a short time before, have worked long and hard to save the very same person's life following a previous attempt; in this situation, it is perceived as the ultimate act of ingratitude.

Nurses may therefore approach suicidal patients with a somewhat mixed and conflicting personal set of attitudes and emotions. This being so, they must attempt to recognize and identify these attitudes and emotions prior to counselling suicidal patients, lest they interfere with the development of the counselling relationship necessary to help a patient through to an appreciation of the value of living. For the nurse as counsellor, just as for any other counselling situation, it is essential that an atmosphere of trust is developed with the patient which will allow the issue of responsibility to be raised in a sensitive and caring way. In the case of a suicidal patient, it is essential that the issue of responsibility is raised since exploring the patient's ambivalence is the key to the successful resolution of suicidal intent (Geldard, 1989, p. 140).

Just as nurses may experience anger in response to suicidal patients, so the patients themselves may also be feeling angry. Research in abnormal psychology has identified anger as an important determinant of the wish to commit suicide, but it is anger directed internally towards the self rather than anger directed outwards to some other person or object. It is important, therefore, when approaching the counselling of a suicidal patient, to consider and explore the possibility that the patient is manifesting inward-directed anger, to look at the reasons for this anger, and to attempt to deal with it in an open manner. Exploring the reasons for a suicide wish or a failed attempt in terms of anger may be helpful in allowing the patient to confront some of the feelings behind the action. Sensitive and caring exploration of the possibility of suicide as a form of self-punishment may provide the patient with insights into their own intents and actions which may never have been faced. The use of such exploration to allow the resolution of old guilts, misdeeds of the past, or present uncertainties of self-worth and self-esteem, when applied by skilled counsellors, is a highly effective way to deal with a suicidal patient.

Of course, suicidal behaviour may also be a way of punishing others. Some may choose to end their lives as a means of punishing a close, significant other for not caring enough or for failing to comply with a set of (perhaps) impossible demands for attention. Counselling in this instance is directed towards manipulative behaviour, but requires very careful clinical judgement as to the seriousness of the suicidal intent and the rationality of the reasons underlying it.

The reactions of nurses to patients brought into hospital immediately following a suicide attempt are crucial. A cold, judgemental response to a teenage girl who has overdosed may merely confirm, in her mind at least, that suicide was the best option after all. By contrast, a sensitive and caring approach, with appropriate reflection of feelings and content, may go some way to reassuring the ambivalent teenager that living is not such a bad outcome.

Management of a suicidal patient, or of a patient who has made an unsuccessful attempt, requires care and caution. Nurses cannot forget that their own pre-existing attitudes and values regarding life and its preservation will enter into the process which guides their response to the patient. Moreover, suicidal intent or attempt constitutes a life threatening condition no less potentially terminal than heart attack or cancer. Whatever the nurse's attitudes and values, a suicidal patient must be taken seriously, carefully monitored, skilfully counselled and at all times considered as a risk. Failure to do this may place the patient in even further danger. Counselling of suicidal patients may well require counselling skills of a very high order, and will certainly be a time-consuming activity. Much of this work will, therefore, be undertaken by purpose trained counsellors, whether clinical psychologists or other mental health professionals, and the nurse's primary role when looking at the counselling needs of suicidal patients might well be one of monitoring, talking and then referring. As always, however, nurses are likely to be the people in most direct and continuing contact with suicidal patients, and their skills in identifying potential problems, and in coordinating the availability of counselling services, are crucial ones.

Patients in Pain

Pain is the ubiquitous companion to illness or injury, and for nurses in clinical practice it is an inescapable reality of daily working life. Patients in pain experience and express a unique distress, based not only on the physical sensation but also on the fear for life and for the continued physical integrity of the person which pain carries with it. The management of a patient in pain is hampered by the medical reality that in some cases there is little that may be done to physically diminish the magnitude of the pain sensation. Pain is a neurophysiologically based phenomenon, taking signals from tissue damaged by injury or the existence of some pathological process and transforming these signals, after complex central nervous system processing, into a subjective experience. It therefore has biological and cognitive (interpretive) elements, both of which may be mobilised in the task of pain management.

The use of counselling or psychological strategies for pain management takes two forms. The first of these attempts to reduce the intensity
of the pain itself. While most medical settings rely on the pharmacological control of pain through the use of analgesics and, occasionally,
on the use of electrophysiological or surgical procedures in extreme and
chronic cases, there are a number of developing psychological strategies
which have use in pain management. Relaxation strategies have been
used effectively with patients in pain, particularly where the pain has a
muscular component, as have strategies based on electromyographic
biofeedback (see Chapter 4). Strategies facilitating the redirection of
attention away from the site of the pain (for example, hypnosis) have
also been used, though the evaluation of their effectiveness remains in its
early stages. Perhaps the most broadly useful of all have been strategies
arising from cognitive techniques, where patients are encouraged to re-
evaluate the sensation of pain in the context of the whole range of
competing stimuli existing in their environments. Peck & Love (1986)
present a clear account of the basic strategies currently used in the
psychological management of pain. It needs to be emphasized, however,
that these are largely specialist skills requiring appropriate technical
training, and are not therefore likely to be brought into use during the
course of routine nursing practice. Nurses, none the less, should know
that such strategies and approaches exist so that they are fully aware of
the services which might be offered to their patients by other professionals within the hospital environment.

The other psychological approach to pain management is more general. Patients in pain are typically also in considerable psychological
distress, as we have said above, and the use of general counselling skills
with these patients has been demonstrated to be beneficial, at least from
the viewpoint of their overall coping. Patients in pain require empathic
listening so that they are not left with the impression (rightly or otherwise) that those tending to their purely medical needs neither understand
nor care about their psychological needs. The simple act of sitting, if
only briefly, with patients in chronic, severe pain, and listening in a
caring and empathic way, may establish or reinforce the view for these
patients that at least there is understanding of the situation. In this
capacity, the nurse as counsellor need not take an active role, or one in
which technical advice must be given, but may simply assume the role of
the listener, reassuring and being part of a therapeutic relationship which
allows the patient to work through the torment of pain. There is good
evidence that such basic counselling may go further than just alleviating
psychological distress, acting as well actually to reduce the level of self-
reported pain. In view of their daily contact with patients in pain, nurses
have a unique potential to fulfil this role.

The Role of the Nurse as Counsellor

It is important to recognize that there are realistic limits to the degree to which nurses are able to take on the role of counsellor. In the first place, few nurses receive sufficient training in counselling to allow them to be involved in a large amount of formal one to one counselling. Second, given the range of duties that nurses are required to undertake, there is often insufficient time for them to engage in lengthy or ongoing counselling with any one patient. This is not to say, however, that the nurse's role as a counsellor is not important. On the contrary, it is of enormous importance. Nurses will be in close contact with patients suffering from a range of disorders, and their psychological approach to the care and attention they give these patients will be a vital element in their recovery. Nurses' counselling skills are, therefore, a necessary component to ensuring that patients receive the quality of care essential for that recovery to take place.

As stressed in the sections on handling angry, grieving and suicidal patients as well as patients in pain, nurses are part of an interconnecting web of trained helping professionals, and as such appropriate referrals to other helpers is a necessary part of the nurses' job. The development of referral networks is therefore an important component of the provision and coordination of counselling help to patients.

Summary and Conclusions

In this chapter, we have attempted to outline the basic qualities of the nurse as counsellor. It was suggested that counselling is about listening rather than active, technical intervention, and that attention to feelings is a crucial skill for helpers to acquire, along with appropriate reflecting, questioning, summarizing and confronting skills. Apart from general counselling skills, attention was given to the handling of specific types of patients which nurses are likely to be required to work with. A lengthy example of training patients in progressive relaxation methods was also given, since the broad application of this will be covered in further chapters. While the technical and time limits of nurses as counsellors were noted, their crucial position as the most immediate contact which patients have was suggested to underscore the centrality of their role both as provider and coordinator of counselling services to their patients.

References/Reading List

Bohart, A.C. & Todd, J. (1988). *Foundations of Clinical and Counseling Psychology*. New York: Harper & Row.

Brammer, L.M. & Shostrom, E.L. (1977). *Therapeutic Psychology: Fundamentals of Counseling and Psychotherapy*, 3rd edition. Englewood Cliffs, New Jersey: Prentice-Hall.

Brammer, L.M., Shostrom, E.L. & Abrego, P.J. (1989). *Therapeutic Psychology: Fundamentals of Counseling and Psychotherapy*, 5th edition. Englewood Cliffs, New Jersey: Prentice-Hall.

Brown, J.H. & Brown, C.S. (1977). *Systematic Counseling: A Guide for the Practitioner*. Champaign, Illinois: Research Press.

Corey, G. (1986). *Theory and Practice of Counseling and Psychotherapy*. Belmont, California: Brooks/Cole.

Corsini, R.J. (1979). *Current Psychotherapies*. Itasca, Illinois: F.E. Peacock.

Corsini, R.J. & Wedding, D. (1989). *Current Psychotherapies*, 4th edition. Itasca, Illinois: F.E. Peacock.

Frank, J.D. (1961). *Persuasion and Healing*. Baltimore: John Hopkins Press.

Fritz, P.A., Russel, C.G., Wilcox, E.M. & Shirk, F.I. (1984). *Interpersonal Communication in Nursing: An Interactionist Approach*. Norwalk, Connecticut: Appleton-Century-Crofts.

Geldard, D. (1989). *Basic Personal Counselling*. New York: Prentice-Hall.

Gilligan, C. (1982). *In a Different Voice*. Cambridge, Massachusetts: Harvard University Press.

Gilliland, B.E. & James, R.K. (1988). *Crisis Intervention Strategies*. Belmont, California: Brooks/Cole.

Gilliland, B.E., James, R.K. & Bowman, J.T. (1989). *Theories and Strategies in Counselling and Psychotherapy*, 2nd edition. Englewood Cliffs, New Jersey: Prentice-Hall.

Gottman, J.M. & Leiblum, S.R. (1974). *How to do Psychotherapy and How to Evaluate it*. New York: Holt, Rinehart & Winston.

Hopson, B. (1978). Counselling in work settings. In P.B. Warr (ed.), *Psychology at Work*. Middlesex: Penguin.

Moursund, J. (1990). *The Process of Counselling and Therapy*. Englewood Cliffs, New Jersey: Prentice-Hall.

Nelson-Jones, R. (1983). *Practical Skills: A Psychological Skills Approach for the Helping Professions and for Voluntary Counsellors*. London: Holt, Rinehart & Winston.

Novaco, R.W. (1975). *Anger Control*. Lexington, Massachusetts: Heath Books.

Peck, C. & Love, A. (1986). Chronic pain. In N.J. King & A. Remenyi (eds), *Health Care: A Behavioural Approach* (pp. 133–144). Sydney: Grune & Stratton.

Prochaska, J.D. (1979). *Systems of Psychotherapy: A Transtheoretical Analysis.* Homewood, Illinois: The Dorsey Press.

Tschudin, V. (1982). *Counselling Skills for Nurses.* London: Bailliere Tindall.

U'Ren, R.C. (1980). *The Practice of Psychotherapy: A Guide for the Beginning Therapist.* New York: Grune & Stratton.

4
Stress, Illness and Nursing Practice

Stress: Descriptions and Definitions

Stress is one of the most widely used concepts in the fields of psychology and psychosocial medicine, and its usage by lay people is even more widely spread. It arises in all kinds of contexts to imply an extraordinary pressure or challenge placed on the individual either from sources outside (most typically) or from internal conflicts, confusions and concerns. Stress is commonly held to be ubiquitous: no one escapes it at some stage or another. A minority of people are unfortunate enough to experience it more often than others, and rarely, though dramatically, a small few suffer from an almost continuous state of stress over a long period of time.

The presence of stress may be noted by those external to the sufferer. It is not uncommon to hear someone described, in lay conversation, by the words: 'She needs gentle treatment and a lot of consideration right now; she is under a lot of stress'. This, of course, implies not only the condition of stress but also some of its consequences, both for the sufferer and for those around her. But equally commonly, it seems, people are now applying the word stress to themselves in order to describe and explain (both to themselves and to others) an unusual state of emotional disquiet, a vague and unaccounted for feeling of physical unwellness or an atypical period during which there is an apparent failure of normally expected coping strategies.

More importantly, however, in the past few decades there has been a burgeoning in the more or less technical use of stress as an explanatory concept in the health sciences. This has been evident on three broad levels of explanation. On the most general, the notion of stress seems more and more to be invoked to account for the unaccountable appearance of symptoms when all reasonable medical investigation fails to provide a biological explanation. On an intermediate level, the presence of stress seems increasingly to be seen as a vulnerability factor, making the appearance of many symptoms and illnesses, themselves not primarily due to stress, more likely than if stress were absent. Finally, and most specifically, there is now a large and still accumulating body of scientific evidence implicating stress, variously conceptualized and measured, either as a causal or contributory factor in the genesis and precipitation of a large range of physical illnesses affecting systems such as the cardiovascular or gastrointestinal systems and the immune system. The concept of stress has, in other words, achieved widespread usage both in the health sciences and lay communities.

Yet definitions of stress remain varied and unclear, and it might sometimes be thought that stress has as many meanings as there are people using the concept. It is often held, especially by those naive in the area, that stress is composed entirely of events and circumstances external to the person, and largely beyond personal control. People are said to be 'facing stress', 'under stress' or 'subject to stress'. This conceptualization of stress emphasizes the environment and essentially discounts the role of the individual. People are seen to be helpless victims of fate or circumstance, passive recipients of external adversity.

The external environment, however, is only part of the story. Stress may only be considered to exist if it is *experienced* by the individual, and it is the experiential component of stress which is perhaps the most interesting, both from psychological and medical perspectives. Given that according to the overall concept of stress, events external to the individual are distinct from those occurring within, it has become common to distinguish these by separate terms.

To take first things first, aspects of the environment which a person encounters, and which may challenge, threaten or pose a potential danger to that person, are termed *stressors*. Stressors may come in many shapes and forms. They may consist of environmental conditions, completely physical in origin, objectively defined and accurately measurable, such as intense heat or cold, excessively loud noise or unacceptably high levels of pollutants in the air. Physical stressors, or at least the potential for them, form the essence of the biosphere in which we all live. For the most part, we are able to protect ourselves from their major impact, typically by the use of other physical means. In other words, we have the capacity, by and large, to create artificial but largely protective physical environments if the natural one becomes too noxious in one way or another. The simple act of turning on a heater creates an artificial environment which serves a protective function.

Within the context of modern medicine, however, stressors of a psychosocial nature are considered more salient to the understanding of stress and illness, and assume a greater prominence than physical stressors, both theoretically and quantitatively. Psychosocial stressors encompass the entire breadth of short term events and longer term situations arising from interactions which individuals have with their interpersonal, social and work environments (we will discuss in more detail further on the nature and presentation of psychosocial stressors). It should be clear from this description that encounters with psychosocial stressors are inescapable consequences of even the most ordinary lifestyles.

Of course, as we shall see later, the impact of any given stressor on different people may vary dramatically. The individual impact of stressors (measured by the magnitude of a person's response to a stressor) is neither objectively determined nor consistent across people. Information conveyed to the person by any given stressor is largely sensory, and its meaning must be arrived at not simply from its nature but also, to a very considerable extent, from the relationship it bears to information already contained within the person's memory. The impact of a stressor is, therefore, determined by individual interpretation of the meaning of the stressor, constructed within personal, contextual frameworks. An *interpretive* component, therefore, forms the next step in the sequence of events making up the stress process.

Once an individual interprets the sensory information contained within an encountered stressor, that individual is ready for the organization and initiation of the final or *responsive* component of the sequence. This component may be divided into two separate but interconnected parts, one being alterations to the psychological equilibrium of the individual and the other alterations to the individual's physiological equilibrium. Physiological disequilibrium typically shows itself as a heightened level of arousal within both the central and autonomic nervous systems; psychological disequilibrium is typically seen as a state of agitation, unrest, hyper-alertness and apprehension (the word *anxiety*, as we shall see in the next chapter, is sometimes used to convey the feeling associated with this state).

Clearly, the *experiential* component of stress has now also been reached and the individual recognizes the existence of stress by the experience of distress. The experience of stress is not pleasant. At best, it involves the recognition of undue pressure or of a transient failure to cope as well as one might expect or at a level achieved in the past. At worst, it may be signalled by both physical and emotional pain, and by the conviction that the body, or at least parts of it, is seriously disordered or compromised in its function.

The complete sequence of stages and events comprising the process of stress, from stressor to experience, may be seen in Figure 4.1 and, as this shows, there is a simple invariance to the sequence. The development of this sequence, or model of stress, owes much to the work of the physiologist Hans Selye, the physician Lennart Levi and the psychologist Richard Lazarus. Each in his turn has added materially to our understanding of the concept of stress, and we will turn to their particular

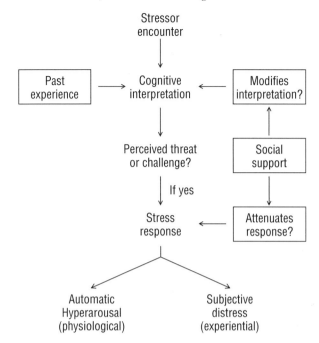

Figure 4.1   *Sequence of stages and events comprising the process of stress*

contributions later in this chapter as the components of stress are discussed in greater detail.

However, even though we now have a structure from which to understand the notion of stress and its importance for human health and illness, we have still not yet provided a formal definition of the concept. As we stated at the outset, this is not easy since the word stress conveys many meanings to many people, either those engaged in its investigation or those having the misfortune to experience it. Recourse to a medical dictionary (in this instance, *The Oxford Concise Medical Dictionary*, 2nd edition, 1987) provides a very general definition when it says that stress is '. . . any factor that threatens the health of the body or has an adverse effect on its functioning . . .' (p. 593). A psychological dictionary (the *Penguin Dictionary of Psychology*, 1985) is somewhat more precise when it defines stress as:

1.   Generally, any force that when applied to a system causes some significant modification of its form, usually with the connotation that the modification is a deformation or distortion.

2.   A state of psychological tension produced by the kinds of forces alluded to in 1 above . . . (pp. 736 to 737).

Neither of these definitions, however, addresses the sequential, process-like nature of stress that we have described briefly above. The following definition, which is really a composite of many attempts to describe and define the concept, has therefore been constructed to encompass the real nature of stress. Thus, for the purposes of this chapter, stress will be defined as: *The collective response, physiological, emotional and behavioural, which is both evident and experienced when a relatively unprepared individual encounters an environment which poses a potential threat, challenge or danger.* This definition carries with it the three components of the process of stress outlined above, namely the *stressor* (environmental) component, the *interpretive* component, and the *responsive/experiential* component. Each of these components will be discussed in further detail as the chapter progresses.

Traditional Psychosomatic Reasoning

The idea that external pressures of a psychosocial kind, or intense emotional reactions to these, may exert a profound influence on the functioning of the body, either in the short or long term, is not new. The Greek physician Hippocrates (around 200 BC) is reported to have said to his students:

> Let no one persuade you to cure the headache until he has first given you his soul to be cured. For this is the great error of our day in the treatment of the human body, that physicians separate the soul from the body.

Through the centuries there has been a consistent recognition among physicians that the mind, the thoughts it processes and the emotions it gives rise to have strongly influenced the health and well-being of the body. In the seventeenth century, the British physician Archer wrote:

> The observation I have made in practice of physick these several years hath confirmed me in this opinion, that the original, or cause, of most mens and womens sickness, disease and death is first, some great discontent which brings a habit of sadness of mind . . .

Some organs of the body, in particular, have been traditionally seen to interact closely with the mind; the heart, for example, was considered the source of the emotional life for many centuries, and while science has led to the adoption of other views in more recent times, the heart continues in literature to be held responsible for greed and malice, sadness and joy, and fear. It was the philosophers and not the physicians, however, who maintained the major part of the historical debate on the psychosomatic nexus, commonly referred to as the mind–body argument in philosophical works.

It was not until around the turn of the twentieth century that the psychosomatic relationship was formalized in medicine, within the context of systematic, biopsychosocial reasoning. This can be rightly attributed to the work of Sigmund Freud and the advent of psychoanalytic theory. Freud conceived of indivisible associations between the mind and the body, and many of his detailed case reports sought to explain quite dramatic physical symptoms, often involving total loss of sensory or motor function, in terms of disturbances of psychological function. In their historic and pioneering work *Studies in Hysteria* published in 1895, Breuer & Freud argued that psychological events and processes, usually buried within the unconscious, could under certain circumstances be symbolically expressed as bodily symptoms and dysfunctions, the nature and location of the expression giving some clue to the meaning of the underlying psychological event. This systematic approach to the psychosomatic relationship, based as it was on a convincing and coherent body of theory and, at least, 'observational data', signalled the beginning of a concerted effort, over the past 90 or so years, towards a fuller and more precise understanding of the real influence of psychological processes on biological functioning in humans. We will now look at some of the landmarks in this effort.

Intrapsychic Conflicts and Bodily Symptoms

For many in the Freudian and neo-Freudian schools, the psychological basis for bodily symptoms was to be found in the existence of intrapsychic conflicts, in which an unconscious urge was at odds with patterns of conscious, socialized behaviour. Karl Abraham, a one-time devotee of Freud, published in 1927 a formulation for the development of intrapsychic conflicts. In this view, Abraham suggested that unconscious 'drives' arising from biological needs (oral and anal) had the potential to generate conflict by competing for expression with more mature and socially complex behaviours. This resulted at times in the symbolic representation of the conflict as symptoms in areas of the body linked to the nature of the conflict. For example, when the unconscious need for oral gratification, arising from early childhood developmental experiences, comes face to face in adulthood with the need to exercise strong social control over the process of eating (in short, manners), this may result in a conflict which becomes expressed in the physical symptoms of anorexia or bulimia nervosa. Groddeck, another theorist in the psychoanalytic tradition, was even more encompassing in his proclamation that every physical illness could be seen as a symbolic representation of some deep and unresolved conflict lying within the unconscious. As the contemporary psychosomatic theorist Lipowski has pointed out, however, such far-ranging speculation did not meet with completely unqualified acceptance.

Psychosomatic Disease Specificity

While conflict theory was not totally dismissed as an explanatory concept in psychosomatic medicine, however, it was married to a newer and developing concept, that of *disease specificity*, to provide a more complete understanding of the role which psychological factors could play in initiating physical symptoms. In the 1940s and early 1950s, deriving their evidence exclusively from psychoanalytic interviews with patients suffering from a variety of physical illnesses, both Flanders Dunbar and Franz Alexander advanced the view that there was a direct and unique relationship between the specific nature or source of the intrapsychic conflict and the emergent physical symptoms, such that the existence of a particular conflict would give rise to one, and only one, illness or set of symptoms. Much of the evidence for this conclusion, as we have said, could be traced to the results of long and detailed psychoanalyses with a very small and limited sample of individuals diagnosed as physically ill but lacking an identified physical or pathological cause. Evidence gained this way does not meet with ready acceptance within the context of contemporary, empirically based psychology.

A novel approach was, however, put forward by those experimenting in the early 1950s with the technique of hypnosis when, using hypnotic suggestion to induce conflict states in normal subjects, reminiscent of those conflicts identified by the work of Dunbar and of Alexander, biological associations between at least some of these states and the physical signs and symptoms they were believed to underlie were able to be demonstated. Symptoms of *urticaria* were found, for example, to be associated with a conflict between feelings of mistreatment and the supressed need for revenge. The experience of *nausea and vomiting* was seen in response to a conflict between regret over a past act or misdeed and the realization that it could never be corrected. Work such as this has added some credibility to the disease specificity view, and while it has, in recent times, been the subject of strong, empirically based criticism, there are some, particularly in the psychoanalytic tradition, who continue to defend it, if only on intuitive grounds. However, the greatest problem arising from theories based on notions of intrapsychic conflict, specific or otherwise, is that they are largely untestable by the scientific method. Concepts are not easily translated into measurable constructs and the methodologies available to test hypotheses derived from such constructs are limited. Acceptance of much of this evidence is, therefore, is essentially an act of faith.

The Physiological Contribution

The contributions of physiology to our understanding of the link between psychological factors and illness has been invaluable in providing a firm scientific foundation to the área. As far back as 1833, Beaumont reported gross changes in the external appearance of the gastric mucosa in response to emotional states, in a man in whom an accident had exposed the structure. In 1920, Walter Cannon described the pattern of physiological responses to be seen when the organism, whether human or otherwise, was subjected to extreme challenge of one kind or another. Cannon wrote that during times of *emergency*, whether from physical or social causes, the organism responded with a generally heightened level of physical activity in a range of body systems including the cardiovascular, gastrointestinal and musculoskeletal systems. These responses were presumed to originate from a single, glandular source and to serve the purpose of maximizing the biological potential of the organism adaptively to face the emergency. The survival value of this biological mechanism, which has become known as the *flight/fight* response, is widely recognized across the biopsychosocial disciplines.

The basic concepts of Cannon's work formed the background for a systematic and cogent view of the psychosomatic relationship put forward by Hans Selye. Based on past work, and on his own clinical observations of the physiological responses of men subjected by the circumstance of war to extreme physical stressors, Selye commenced a long and detailed series of clinical and laboratory studies aimed at exploring the patterns and causes of physiological responses to externally imposed stressors. As a result of this work, Selye described the *General Adaptation Syndrome* (GAS), in which exposure to a stressor elicits a three-stage response in an invariant order. The first of these stages, Selye called the *alarm reaction*; in this stage, the organism is activated by the immediate threat posed to it. The pituitary gland liberates adrenocorticotrophic hormone (ACTH), and this stimulates the adrenal gland to produce a general state of activation within the autonomic nervous system. The second stage, which Selye called the *resistance stage*, uses the physiological changes brought about by the alarm reaction to equip the organism to face and overcome its state of threat. Finally, in the *exhaustion stage*, which occurs only if the resistance stage is prolonged and the threat is not overcome, physiological resources for activation become depleted and the organism enters an area of risk of disease or death.

Indeed, many studies with laboratory animals have shown that death from demonstrable tissue pathology in several body systems, notably the cardiovascular and gastrointestinal systems, may be the direct result of prolonged exposure of the organism to unavoidable stressors. It is well known now that animals placed in environments which force them to endure unavoidable stressors over extended periods of time (rats in excessively crowded colonies or monkeys facing unpredictable, painful electric shock are two examples) have a higher mortality rate than genetically identical animals living in their normal environments. Moreover, the cause of death is frequently found to be either coronary occlusion and resulting myocardial infarction, or gastric ulceration and massive bleeding. While this evidence does not directly show a cause–effect relationship between the occurrence of a stressor and premature death, the coincidental evidence is persuasive at the very least.

More recent work, for example that of Levi and his colleagues in the 1970s and 1980s, has benefited from the availability of measures of physiological function far more sensitive and sophisticated than could have been conceived of in Selye's time. Moreover, Levi's creative theories in stress and disease have been able to draw on elaborate psychosocial conceptualizations of the human environment. As such, they have added enormously to our understanding of the psychosomatic relationship. The importance of Selye's work is, however, underscored by the observation that elements of the GAS are still to be seen in more modern and more complex models of the psychosocial influence on physiological functioning.

Contributions from Learning Theory

Parallel with developments in the physiology of adaptation over the past 90 years, psychological laboratories were producing a growing body of experimental evidence on the role of learning in the alteration of physiological functioning. Pavlov's concept of classical conditioning, as already outlined in Chapter 1, may be seen as the forerunner of this activity. Pavlov was able to show that dogs could be taught to produce involuntary physiological responses, salivation and gastric secretion, on the presentation of stimuli quite unrelated to the biological production of these responses. By continually pairing presentations of an unconditioned stimulus (food, for example) with a completely unrelated conditioned stimulus (a sound, a shape or a colour), the biologically based unconditioned response (salivation or gastric secretion), which initially occurred only as a direct biological consequence of the appearance of the unconditioned stimulus, in time became a conditioned response which could be evoked by the appearance of the conditioned stimulus alone. This work provided the theoretical basis, at least, for the view that the organism is capable of learning maladaptive physiological responses by the deliberate or fortuitous pairing of innocuous and biologically active stimuli. It is thought that the physiological effects of the biologically active stimulus may be maintained, perhaps to the organism's detriment, long after withdrawal of that stimulus, so long as exposure to the (initially) innocuous stimulus occurs from time to time.

Within the field of learning theory, as we have shown in Chapter 1, the initial interest in Pavlov's model of learning was, for many years, overshadowed by the advent of *operant* or *instrumental conditioning*, heralded by the work of Thorndike in the first decades of the twentieth century and systematized by Skinner in the 1930s and later. However, while operant conditioning provided a highly relevant framework for the understanding of overt behaviours, it was not considered to have any bearing on physiological functioning until the imaginative work of Miller and his colleagues in the 1950s and 1960s showed that physiological functioning could be brought under individual control by the operation of reward and punishment.

In a series of widely acclaimed experiments, Miller and his colleagues showed that laboratory rats could learn to raise or lower both heart rate and blood pressure by the researchers reinforcing initially random variations in these functions with short bursts of electrical stimulation to the 'pleasure centre' of the brain. In a typical study, rats were anaesthetized to allow the implantation of stimulating electrodes into an histologically distinct area of their forebrains. It was known that electrical stimulation of this area acted as a powerful reinforcer in experiments adopting the operant conditioning paradigm. Implantation of transducers to allow accurate measurement of cardiovascular function (heart rate and blood pressure) was also achieved during the surgery. On regaining consciousness, the animals were placed into a restraining apparatus which severely restricted free movement, and cardiovascular function was monitored by the researchers.

At first, small and quite random variations in the cardiovascular function of interest to the particular experiment (heart rate or blood pressure) were reinforced by electrical stimulation to the 'pleasure centre' through the implanted stimulating electrodes. After several trials of this, however, it was found that the animals were able to alter their heart rates or blood pressures in the direction in which change had been reinforced almost immediately they entered the restraining apparatus. Rats reinforced for decreases in heart rate, for example, were noted to show this soon after coming into the experimental situation. Those, by contrast, reinforced for increases in blood pressure, showed this response upon entering the experimental situation. Moreover, the cardiovascular response within the experimental situation complied with all the rules of learning set out by Skinner in his account of operant conditioning. This work not only provided the explanation as to why aberrant patterns of physiological functioning may become ingrained through learning, and lead to the formation of physical pathology, but also laid the foundation for the treatment of physiological dysfunction by learning procedures using the technique of biofeedback (see later in this chapter).

Transfer of Interest from Individual to Environment

Much of the early work bearing on our understanding of the complex but self-evident relationship between psychological events and physical symptoms focused attention squarely onto the individual. It was the person whose 'maladaptive' development was seen to produce intrapsychic conflict leading, in turn, to the appearance of symptoms. Disturbed patterns of 'mental' functioning within the person, and not the environmental context in which 'mental' functioning developed or existed, were held responsible for any psychosomatic relationship in evidence at any time.

It was not until the 1960s, with an upsurge of interest in the theoretical basis of stress and its role in physical ill health, that a systematic concern for the possible role of the social environment became apparent. Selye's work had certainly shown that stressors to be found in the physical environment could, by way of the GAS, exert a profound influence on risk of illness. Physical stressors are, however, reasonably easily defined and measured, making the investigation of their relationships with illness a comparatively simple task. Psychosocial stressors, by contrast, pose a somewhat more difficult problem, both conceptually and for measurement. None the less, the psychosocial environment is sufficiently important from the standpoint of stress and illness to merit detailed attention.

Characteristics of the Noxious Social Environment

Psychosocial stressors are widely disparate in their nature and origins. They range in onset and duration from acute, brief and strictly transient *events* arising from fortuitous encounters, through to involvement in protracted, largely open-ended *situations* arising from complex psychological or social transactions over which the individual may have some personal control, albeit limited.

Workers in the field of mental health and, to some extent, internal medicine, have long recognized the role which the social environment may play in the precipitation and course of illness. For the greater part of this time, however, investigation of the role was relegated to casual observations of occasions in which the environment was seen to influence the onset or course of an illness, and to conclusions drawn from these interesting but unsupportable data. Indeed, it was only in the early sixties, with the work of Holmes & Rahe, that systematic attempts were made to define the characteristics of the social environment (at least from a limited perspective), quantify their impact on the individual and test statistically the relationship between this impact and both present and future illness.

In 1967, Holmes & Rahe published the first list of *stressors* or *life events*, in which they attempted to characterize in a succinct manner those aspects of the social environment which might, by their impact, tax the individual sufficiently to contribute to illness onset or exacerbate existing illness. The inventory which they used to achieve this, the *List of Recent Experiences*, was a list of 43 commonly experienced life events or situations which might occur to anyone at some stage in their lives. Events or situations ranged from the seemingly trivial, like getting a parking ticket, to events of undeniable impact on most people, like the death of a close relative or friend.

Recent research has added considerably to the content of life event inventories and the nature of the items has been refined to ensure inclusion both of events and situations. An extensive inventory designed for use in a major study of the effects of the social environment on the development of neurotic illness, undertaken and reported by Henderson, Byrne & Duncan-Jones in 1981, serves to illustrate the scope of modern life event measurement inventories. This particular instrument, with 73 items, covered the following life event or recent experience categories:

Illness, injury or accident
Bereavement
Pregnancy or childbirth
Changes in relationships
Separations (interpersonal)
Changes in living conditions
Education
Work situation
Financial situation
Legal difficulties
Disappointments
Continuous worry or stress

In the early days of life event research, the methodology was simple. Subjects, whether patients, others with problems or normal persons, were given a printed inventory of life events and asked to indicate those events (or situations) which had actually happened to them in a given period of time. This time frame was typically a one year period prior to the collection of life events data. The frequency of life event exposure or encounter, simply measured as the number of life events indicated as experienced in the given time period, was said to relate to the probability of illness in the near future. As a research technique, however, this proved too simplistic an approach to tap the somewhat complex associations between stress and illness. This approach ignored that component of the stress concept which underscores the importance of the interpretations which individuals place upon those events or situations befalling them.

Holmes & Rahe suggested that life events or situations acquired their pathogenic impact by way of the extent to which any given event or situation demanded change or adjustment. They therefore attempted to attach a numerical index to each item in their 43 event list, to indicate the extent to which that event (or situation) demanded personal adjustment or life change. They did this by assigning an entirely arbitrary 'life change' score of 500 to the life event marriage and then instructed a sample of healthy subjects to give scores above or below 500 to each of the other 42 items to reflect the degree to which these would demand life change or adjustment of the 'average person'. By averaging responses over their subject sample, they arrived at a set of weightings which quantified the impact of life events (or situations). The resultant set of averaged weightings, used in association with the List of Recent Experiences, they called the *Social Readjustment Rating Scale*. This produced a marked improvement in the methodology available to studies of life events and illness, since it took the quantification of life events (and situations) from a simple frequency account of occurrences to a single, numerical index of the impact of life events in a given time. Now, researchers were not only able to obtain counts of life events (or situations) but could attach impact weightings to these, sum the impact weightings over the number of reported life events and present a number indicating life event impact which took account of the varying nature of the life events (or situations) themselves.

The work of Holmes and Rahe in identifying life change as the mediating construct of life event impact, and their construction of scales to measure this, must be considered seminal in the description of the noxious social environment. More recently, however, interest in the notion of *distress* has overtaken life change as the more prominent mediating construct interposed between life events (or situations) and pathological responses. Still, the basic methodology of identifying personal encounters with life events (or situations) and quantifying their impact by means of weighted scales of life change or distress remains the primary means of characterizing the noxious social environment both for research purposes and, more commonly now, in clinical practice.

Characteristics of the Protective Social Environment

While much of the attention in early studies of illness and the social environment was firmly devoted to what has broadly been termed *adversity*, interest more recently has been given over as much to those aspects of the social environment which might exert a buffering or protective influence in the fact of life events. Within this area, the bulk of work has centred on the identification, specification and measurement of *networks of social support*. As with the area of life events, the published literature abounds with anecdotal accounts and informed speculation regarding the desirability of supportive social networks, both in health and in illness. The advent of systematic research on the nature and usefulness of social networks has, however, been largely restricted to the past two decades.

Over this time, a number of systematic research studies have not only affirmed the value of social networks (sometimes referred to as *social bonds*) in the prevention of psychological symptoms in the face of stress, but have also suggested the importance of absent or impoverished social networks as an independent cause of psychological symptoms. The contribution of the sociologist Brown in Britain perhaps marked the beginnings of this area. He found that in a sample of working class women attending their general practitioners for complaints which were largely psychological in presentation much could be attributed to the presence of significant stressors in their lives. However, those women who reported the absence of social networks, or the impoverishment of those networks available to them, seemed far more vulnerable to the effects of stressor exposure than those for whom a supportive social network was there for use if required.

Henderson and his colleagues, in Australia, took up this work in an effort both to describe in more detail the nature of supportive social networks and to establish the independence of social networks in the cause of symptoms, particularly those of a psychological or neurotic kind. Their work showed that social support could be derived from a range of networks varying in power from close attachments to single individuals, to loose associations with service providers. Drawing on the work of Weiss, this group described six categories of social networks, in descending order of power, as:

1. Attachment — provided by close, affectional relationships giving a sense of sharing and security.
2. Social integration — provided by membership of a group of people holding common interests and values.
3. Opportunity for nurturing — usually arising from the care of children but sometimes of dependent parents or older relatives, providing incentive for continuing activity.
4. Reassurance of personal worth — obtained from relationships promoting self-esteem.
5. Sense of reliable alliance — obtained from the recognition that others are there to help in the face of need or crisis.
6. Help and guidance — in which formal or informal advice and assistance may be sought in the face of specific and usually time-limited demands.

According to Henderson and his colleagues, all individuals have a given, though variable need for support derived from social networks, and could draw on the resources provided by any of these categories, though since they are listed in descending order of importance, it will be clear that networks providing attachment are, for example, more powerful in their capacity to protect in the face of stressors than networks only providing, say, opportunity for nurturance. In practice, it was suggested that most individuals constructed their social support not exclusively from one category or another but from provisions contained in most if not all of the categories. Of course, if deficiencies occurred in one category, they could in principle be counteracted by additional resources to be found in another category. Importantly, individuals do vary in the need or requirement for social support, and the social network cannot be described only in terms of the objective availability of particular kinds of social relationships. It was necessary, therefore, in the measuring instruments devised by Henderson and his colleagues, to have scales not only of availability but also of individual satisfaction with what was available.

Using such scales in a large, general population sample, these workers were able to show that satisfaction with one's social network, at least, protected against the onslaught of stressors. Moreover, it was also evident that conspicuous deficiencies in social networks rendered some people vulnerable to the experience of psychological symptoms, even when stressors were not present in disproportionate numbers. Thus, it is possible to speak of a protective social environment as one abundantly or at least adequately supplied with social resources forming a personal network which may be drawn on in the face of crisis or adversity. It is also possible to describe the characteristics of this social environment and to measure the degree of protection it provides. It is, however, possible as well to note that the absence of a protective social environment may not only be a neutral event, of no consequence except in the face of crisis, but may be in itself a noxious element in the psychosocial matrix within which we all live. Indeed, a simple scan of inventories of life events will confirm that many items, particularly those to do with personal relationships, are in fact characterized by circumstances marking a transition from an adequate to an impoverished social network.

The Stress Reaction

Stressors and their Measurement

The nature of stressors has been outlined above. Briefly, these are events or situations within the individual's psychosocial environment which impact in such a way as to imply danger, threat or challenge. Stressors, or life events as they are sometimes called, take many forms, and lists or inventories of stressors (or life events or recent experiences) vary widely in their coverage, from relatively short lists such as that of Holmes & Rahe to very long and comprehensive lists. It is clear from some of the longer lists that there is much overlap, and it was perhaps the intention of the researchers composing these lists to provide as complete and detailed a coverage as possible of the whole universe of potential stressors, so as to allow subjects in research studies and clinical investigations a 'menu' of stressors from which to describe most adequately their own experiences.

There have, however, been criticisms of the use of self-report instruments in the measurement of stressors. The issue of recall of stressor exposure over time has been called into question, and it has been suggested that accuracy of recall declines with time so that self-reported stressor exposure recalled from about six months ago or more must be doubted for its complete accuracy. It has been suggested that while stressors of considerable importance and magnitude will be remembered with ease and accuracy, stressors of a lesser magnitude, though important at the time of occurrence, may not be remembered nearly so well. Studies have been undertaken to investigate this effect, Typically, they have involved recall of past stressors by a subject, and confirmation of the occurrence of those stressors either by interview with a close relative or friend, or by checks with available records (as may be possible with some captive populations such as long-stay patients). The problem of recall has been documented to some extent but it does not appear to be of a degree which would totally invalidate the bulk of studies relying on self-reported stressor exposure to establish links between stress and illness.

Another factor entering into the debate on recall has to do with the circumstances under which recall is required. Some have suggested that individuals asked to recall stressor experiences during states of emotional distress will, because they are seeking explanations for their distress, recall stressors which did not actually occur, or recall the impact of real stressors as greater than they actually were. There is no evidence for the first of these suggestions. People in states of emotional distress, even when presented with lists of stressors to prompt their memories, have not been shown to be inordinately inaccurate in their recall of personal stressor experiences relative to emotionally stable individuals. The issue of recall of the impact of stressors is somewhat more doubtful though the area requires considerably more systematic investigation before we are able to state with certainty whether or not this poses a particular problem with regard to the accuracy of data already collected.

The Individual Interpretive Process

As we have demonstrated earlier, stressors achieve the large part of their impact on the individual not so much because of their 'objective nature' but because they are interpreted as potentially threatening, dangerous or challenging by the individual. The psychologist Richard Lazarus has been instrumental in establishing the importance and function of the interpretive process. In a series of laboratory experiments, Lazarus was able to show that experimental subjects, chosen for their intelligence and emotional stability, could interpret precisely the same stimulus situation differently according to an *interpretive or cognitive set* established at the beginning of the experiment. His subjects were all exposed to the same stimulus or stressor, a graphic film of a primitive circumcision ceremony. One randomly chosen half of the subjects was told at the outset that the ceremony was of great social importance to those undergoing the ritual and was looked on as a positive event; the other half was told that it was a barbaric ritual involving pain, fear and risk of disease. Measures of the stress response (see later) taken before, during and after the film showed clearly that a positive cognitive set produced a stress response or marginal magnitude whereas a negative cognitive set resulted in a substantial stress response involving both emotional distress and physiological arousal for the subjects in that group.

It is clear, both from experimental and clinical evidence, that individuals do interpret their environments in different ways, and that their responses, both emotional and physiological, are moulded by these interpretations. Obviously, the 'objective nature' of a stressor brings with it some indication of the impact it will have on the individual. The impact of the stressor 'death of a close relative of friend', for example, is likely for most to be a distressing occurrence. It is possible, however, that the circumstances of pain and disability preceding that death may have been far more distressing for those involved, and that the death itself could easily have been interpreted as an event of some relief. The point to be taken is that factors far broader than the simple description of a stressor must be considered either in measuring the impact of that stressor or in implying its importance for the individual experiencing it.

Factors Bearing on the Interpretive Process

The manner in which individuals interpret their experience is highly individual specific, as we pointed out earlier. The basis for this specificity lies with a range of factors which shape perceptions of life events. The most global of these is individual personality.

Possession of the personality attribute of *neuroticism*, defined as instability of personality, has in fact been shown to influence life events experience in two ways. First, those with the attribute of neuroticism (which may easily be measured using a standard questionnaire known as the Eysenck Personality Questionnaire) appear to encounter more life events than those not so characterized by the attribute. Second, possession of neuroticism seems to accentuate the interpretation of life events in such a way that they are perceived by these people as more dangerous, threatening or challenging than they are by those without the attribute. This is not surprising since research into the concept and meaning of neuroticism suggests that it has much to do with coping failure or the incapacity of individuals to deal adaptively with those life events they encounter.

The personality attribute of *locus of control* (LOC), too, seems to influence the ways in which life events are interpreted. Locus of control refers to the tendency for individuals to attribute cause to external events, and is typically divided into external LOC, where cause is generally seen to arise from the operation of influences outside the individual, and internal LOC, where cause is attributed to the self. Those with external LOC interpret the life events they encounter as less dangerous, threatening or challenging than those with internal LOC. Once more, this is not surprising, since people who focus on the self take on more personal responsibility for all that happens to them and are less able than others to adopt realistic and balanced views of themselves in proper context.

There is recent evidence that the set of attributes known as the *type A behaviour pattern* (TABP), sometimes incorrectly identified as a personality trait, also influences the rate at which life events are encountered and the manner in which they are interpreted. The TABP consists of a set of behaviours made up of competitiveness, high need for achievement, time urgency, low tolerance for frustration and overt hostility. It has achieved recognition because of the link with risk of coronary heart disease which has been identified by some epidemiological studies. Those with the TABP, as with neuroticism, appear not only to encounter more life events but to interpret those they encounter as more dangerous, threatening or challenging than those without the TABP (so called type B individuals). It has been suggested that the lifestyle arising from possession of the TABP, with its emphasis on achievement, rush and hurry, aggressive competition and self-interest, is eminently suitable to the creation of life events and to the interpretation of each of these as crisis situations.

Past experience and current expectations have also been shown to influence the ways in which individuals interpret life events. Those who expect an event to be personally traumatic in some way or other are more likely to perceive that event in a threatening or challenging way than those adopting a more neutral expectation. Similarly, those who have previously experienced an event, either personally or vicariously, are likely to interpret a future occurrence of that event as more potentially threatening or challenging than those naive to a particular event. There is some evidence of a reverse effect in this respect, with those having experienced a particularly unpleasant event tending to perceive further occurrences of that event as less unpleasant than the initial exposure. This evidence has derived largely from studies in which illness comprises the life event.

The Physiological Response

Life events interpreted as posing potential danger, threat or challenge have a pronounced effect on both the central and peripheral nervous systems. In the immediate term, exposure to a stressor so interpreted results in excitation of the *hypothalamus*, the regulatory portion of the autonomic nervous system within the brainstem. Nerve impulses from the hypothalamus stimulate the *adrenal medulla*, the outer part of the adrenal glands which sit at the top of the kidneys. Stimulation of this organ results in liberation of *catecholamines* (*adrenalin* and *noradrenalin*) which are neurotransmitters; these substances act on organ systems within the body to exert a largely stimulatory effect, commonly termed arousal. Clearly, the anatomy and physiology of this process is complex and beyond the scope of this chapter, but the interested reader will find an excellent account in Hoyenga & Hoyenga (1984). The process has been summarized in Figure 4.2.

At the level of external observation, individuals faced with exposure to life events they interpret as potentially threatening, dangerous or challenging will respond with a range of somatic symptoms engaging all major body systems. The cardiovascular system shows evidence of increased heart rate, diastolic and systolic blood pressure, peripheral

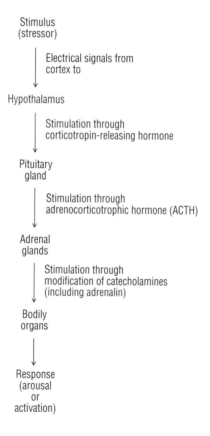

Figure 4.2   *Summary of the physiological response to stress*

vasoconstriction, rapid pulse transit times and redistribution of blood away from visceral organs and into the brain and muscle systems. The gastrointestinal system responds with gastric hypersecretion, increased gut motility and decreased blood flow, producing sensations of gastric uneasiness. Muscles typically increase in tension and ecrine sweat gland activity to both palmar and plantar surfaces is enhanced. In short, the individual is prepared, as we have mentioned earlier, for flight or fight in response to the encountered life event. Regrettably, as we have also pointed out, neither flight nor fight is an appropriate social response for the large majority of physical symptoms arising from this process of arousal, and the final result is usually the experience of physical unease with no obvious outlet for dissipation.

The Psychological Response

Individuals under such conditions of arousal typically report feelings of distress. The emotional state most closely synonymous with distress is that of *anxiety*. Indeed, classical views of anxiety, as we have said earlier, hold that it is no more than the subjective perception of physiological arousal arising from exposure to environmental events. However the origin of the emotional state is seen, whether as an independent consequence of life event exposure or as an accompaniment to physiological arousal, emotional distress provides one of the clearest indications that life events have been encountered and perceived in adverse ways.

There is some debate as to whether exposure to life events is causally responsible, in the long term, for clinical anxiety, or whether it acts merely as a precipitant for the operation of more complex biopsychosocial processes. There is also evidence that long term stress resulting in chronic, environmentally generated anxiety may transform to depression. Thus, the form and natural history of emotional distress following life event exposure is not totally clear. None the less, emotional distress is the first and probably the most important indication of the presence of a noxious social environment.

Stress and Illness

The relevance of the psychological study of stress to the practice of nursing clearly lies with the relationship which stress bears to illness. We will consider some of the evidence documenting this relationship both here and in the following chapter on emotions. Briefly, the links between stress and illness may be examined both with regard to the contribution of the former to the onset of illness, and to the roles stress plays in recovery from illness regardless of the causes of the original onset. The factor which most obviously figures in this set of possible links is that of time. Stress has a well documented acute reaction, manifest, as we have already discussed, both in terms of psychological distress and physiological arousal. In the longer term, however, there is evidence that protracted physiological arousal, encompassing activity in the major neuro-endocrine pathways of autonomic regulation, has the capacity to generate tissue pathology within a wide range of organ systems and biological regulatory processes.

The Acute Reaction

In the immediate term, exposure to environmental stressors results in the combined reaction of emotional distress and autonomic arousal. This in itself can not be seen as illness but as an acute reaction to difficult environmental circumstances. Thus, while the individual may be said to be experiencing acute *distress*, it is essentially time limited and may be expected to disappear on termination of the acute environmental stressor. Some have suggested that the psychological component of this, at least, since it may involve periods of severe mood disorder manifest as anxiety or depression, should be considered as an episode of illness. This very much depends upon the definition one takes of psychological illness, and, certainly, such psychiatric diagnostic systems as the DSM III-R (*Diagnostic and Statistical Manual of the American Psychiatric Association*) would take careful account of acute stress in the diagnosis of a number of psychiatric syndromes. Still, it must be remembered that the brief time frame of the acute reaction limits to a large extent the application of the illness label to a phenomenon which is mainly responsive to external events.

Stress and Tissue Pathology

Most models of stress, including the seminal one of Levi and his colleagues, suggest that if the acute reaction lasts long enough, the cumulative physiological effects of the stress reaction may cause living tissue of various kinds to produce pathological changes. Early observational studies suggested that observable changes to the appearance of the gut could be seen to follow from periods of overt emotional distress. More recently, much evidence has become available to suggest associations between environmental stress and chemical changes which have the potential to create pathology within body tissue. The release of neurotransmitters, for example, might be expected to impact on the cardiovascular system in such a way as to promote damage under periods of extreme or prolonged stress. Similarly, gastric hypersecretion of digestive acids during periods of stress might, if extreme or prolonged, damage the mucosal lining of the gut walls. Immunological changes too have now been shown to follow periods of stress, leading to the speculation that stress may render the body vulnerable to insult from external sources.

There are, however, many unanswered questions regarding the ways in which stress, in the long term, might influence the development of physical pathology. Mechanisms of possible influence are not well understood, and while there is sufficient evidence to suggest very plausible links between stress and tissue pathology, the actual methodology for demonstrating these links is extraordinarily difficult. For clear ethical reasons, experiments cannot be done on living tissue in *situ*, and so much of the evidence must be indirect. Moreover, the time course over which the immediate physiological effects of the stress reaction might be expected to produce tissue pathology is unclear. It is likely to vary with the nature and severity of the stressor situation, the extent of the stress reaction, the nature of the tissue under attack, the general health of the individual and a multitude of other individual-specific factors. Thus, we have much research to do before making definite pronouncements on stress and tissue pathology.

One psychophysiological mechanism which is of interest in this respect, however, is that of *autonomic response specificity*. The psychologist Lacey discovered in the 1950s that while there was a general increase in arousal within organ systems controlled by the autonomic nervous system following a stressful event, one organ system in particular seemed to be maximally responsive to the onset of a stressor. This organ system varied from one individual to another in a way which was consistent and observable but not predictable. Thus, some individuals were cardiovascular responders, and in the face of stress, responded maximally by elevations of heart rate, blood pressure and other haemodynamic functions. Others were found to be gastric responders who, when faced with a stressor, showed gastric hypersecretion and elevations in gut motility. Maximal responding was seen in other organ systems too. Lacey was not able to predetermine from either psychological or physiological information what organ system would respond maximally to stress for any given individual but was able, by careful psychophysiological measurement, to demonstrate consistent autonomic response specificity within single individuals. No explanation for this phenomenon has yet been found though it is assumed that it arises from genetically endowed, constitutional factors.

Its importance for the area of stress and tissue pathology is clear. Individuals showing maximal physiological responsivity to stress in one particular organ system, whatever that may be, could be expected over the course of prolonged stress to sustain most damage to that system, particularly if the nature of the physiological response had pathological potential. Thus, autonomic response specificity might identify organ systems vulnerable to the accumulated effects of stress and, for individuals known to be subject to high levels of stress, focus preventive measures aimed at reducing the subsequent damage. Work in this area is in its infancy but has considerable promise.

Stress and Symptoms

By far and away the strongest evidence linking stress with illness comes from both epidemiological and clinical studies of stress in relation to symptoms. These studies vary considerably in terms of their design (prospective or retrospective), the nature of the stress measures (life event inventories or scales of psychological dysfunction), the manner in which symptom data were collected (self-report or clinical examination), sample sizes, duration of data collection and the nature of the illness or condition under investigation. Each of these factors has a substantial bearing on the reported link between stress and symptoms, not only in so far as the link exists but also with regard to the confidence we may have of the data themselves. None the less, a great deal of persuasive and respectable evidence has become available to suggest that those individuals experiencing stress will also have a higher probability than others of going on to develop symptoms of one kind or another.

Perhaps the seminal work in this area has been that of Rahe and his colleagues working with the Social Readjustment Rating Scale. Their research showed clear associations between accumulations of life events demanding life change and the subsequent onset of diverse symptoms ranging from minor infections and injuries to major life threatening illness such as myocardial infarction (heart attack). Most of the contemporary research has, however, focused on links between stress and symptoms of specific illness events, and among these, certain categories of illness stand out as having stronger established links with stress than others.

Some of the earliest studies of stress and symptoms have focused on the gastrointestinal tract and interest in this area has been enduring. The early but important observations of Wolff and his colleagues laid the foundation for more modern studies linking stress to various kinds of gut disease. In general, current research has divided its attention between studies of environmental stressors in relation to onset, symptoms and course of clinically identified gastrointestinal disease, and studies of stressor exposure in relation to symptoms of biological precursors to gastrointestinal disease.

Data on the former of these vary in the conclusions they allow, but there is now sufficiently persuasive evidence to support the view that individuals exposed to environmental stress suffer a significantly higher rate of both gastric and duodenal ulcers than those not so prone to stress. Much of this work is, however, cross-sectional in nature, and inferences regarding psychological causes of gastrointestinal disease are limited. Two other sources of evidence, both deriving from experimental studies of animals, provide stronger clues to the role of stress in gastrointestinal disease.

It may be shown that animals subjected to difficult or insoluble tasks in the laboratory situation secrete greater quantities of gastric acids, presumed to have an eroding effect on the gastric mucosal tissue, than animals required to perform more neutral tasks. These effects last only as long as the animal is exposed to the stressor (the difficult or insoluble task) and rates of gastric secretion return to normal soon after termination of the stressful situation. Under some experimental situations, however, particularly where exposure to the stressor is prolonged or intense, actual pathological damage to gut tissue may be demonstrated. Brady's work on so-called *executive monkeys* illustrates this well. In his experiment, Brady placed two monkeys side by side in a restraining apparatus such that both were able to receive painful electric shocks. One of the monkeys, the executive monkey, was then trained to recognize a pre-shock cue, a light, which if responded to by the press of a lever, resulted in avoidance of shock both to it and its mate. Animals were run on this apparatus intermittently, for long periods of time, until it was observed, at around the 36th day, that executive monkeys were dying suddenly. Post-mortem examinations revealed the cause of death to be extensive gastric ulceration, a condition which was not found in the non-executive monkeys (those who simply endured the shocks but had no responsibility for controlling them).

The evidence on life event stress and gastrointestinal disease in humans, together with that derived from experimental studies of stress and mechanisms for gastric ulceration in animals, when taken jointly, presents a compelling case for the possible role of psychological factors in diseases of the gut, particularly those to do with erosion of mucosal tissue and ulceration. The executive monkey experiments, while requiring the assumption that imposition of responsibility for control resulted in stress, add considerably to this view.

An area of illness which has received even more attention with regard to stress is that of coronary heart disease. Once again, there is a wealth of evidence that individuals exposed to excessive life event stress are more at risk of clinical coronary heart disease (typically myocardial infarction) than those not so exposed. As with the evidence on gut disease, the retrospective nature of much of this evidence limits its explanatory utility. However, data from three additional areas of investigation strengthen the claim of a link between stress and coronary heart disease quite considerably. People once exposed to catastrophic stressors (war, incarceration in concentration camps, involvement in natural or man-made disasters, for example) appear to have higher subsequent rates of coronary heart disease incidence, sometimes many years after the event, than matched groups of people free from exposure to such catastrophic events. The range of evidence for this effect is extensive and while the studies are methodologically poor, and require cautious interpretation, their volume warrants attention.

Moreover, it can be shown that stressful situations influence some risk factors for coronary heart disease in ways detrimental to the individual. Periods of stress increase blood pressure, at least while the individual is exposed to the stressor, and there is recent evidence that stress may act to elevate blood levels of potentially harmful fats (some fractions of cholesterol), either through dietary regulation or endogenous metabolic means. Thus, risk factor profiles for coronary heart disease may be influenced by the presence of stress, and while this cannot be claimed as a direct effect of stress on the cardiovascular system, its ultimate result of an elevated risk of heart attack is the same.

One of the most prominent areas of investigation in the area of psychological factors and heart disease has been concerned with the influence of the type A behaviour pattern mentioned above. This pattern of behaviour has been shown in many retrospective studies, and several extensive prospective ones, to relate to risk and incidence of coronary heart disease. Traditional views of the TABP would deny any relationship of the behaviour pattern to stress; however, recent work suggests that possession of the TABP both encourages stressful life events and results in states of psychological as well as physical distress. The actual mechanisms through which the TABP influences risk of coronary heart disease are much debated but little understood. These range from possible enhancement of cardiovascular reactivity to environmental stressors, through to a suggestion that those with the TABP deny early symptoms of coronary heart disease, fail to seek medical help or modify their lifestyles soon enough, and thus place themselves at greater risk of coronary morbidity or even mortality. Whatever future investigations tell us, it is likely that illness risk will be mediated by complex neurohormonal mechanisms indicating integral involvement of the central nervous system (see, for example, Byrne & Rosenman, 1990).

Gastrointestinal disease and coronary heart disease provide by no means the only examples of evidence linking stress with illness; they simply provide the clearest account of a patently complex body of evidence. This is an area of rapidly growing research activity and one in which exciting developments may be expected.

Stress and the Recovery/Rehabilitation Process

Stress and Recovery from Illness

It is clearly unlikely that once illness has manifested itself, those stressors which might have contributed to it, or the tendency among some individuals to interpret stressors in challenging or threatening ways, will disappear. Indeed, since illness itself acts as a stressor, it is very probable that the individual will become burdened with at least one more stressor than the load existing prior to illness. Moreover, since a primary stressor such as illness may bring with it a set of secondary stressors such as financial difficulties, family and interpersonal problems, the individual's stressor load is likely to increase considerably as a direct result of illness. Thus, stress during the period of recovery from illness and rehabilitation after it must be considered in the overall program of patient management following illness.

Despite this rationale, the scientific evidence on the influence of stress on recovery and rehabilitation is somewhat sparse. Perhaps the most systematic evidence is to be found for heart attack where it has been shown that those patients experiencing undue and unresolved emotional distress following the initial illness have poorer outcomes, measured in terms of reinfarction, medical complications and return to work, than those adopting a less emotionally traumatic response to their illness. Generally similar results have been shown for patients undergoing renal dialysis, patients recovering from surgery of various kinds and women recovering from difficult childbirth. While the mechanisms explaining this effect are little understood and are likely to vary from one illness type to another, it has been suggested that the mediating effect of arousal within the autonomic nervous system should not be underestimated in considering this process.

More broadly, the effect of stress on outcome after illness may be discussed within the ambit of *abnormal illness behaviour*. The concept of illness behaviour refers to the collection of responses which any individual has to the experience of illness. For the most part, illness behaviour is adaptive and consistent with the nature of the illness, but when such responses are inordinately severe relative to the threat or discomfort of the illness, or where they conflict with activities necessary for recovery and rehabilitation, they are termed abnormal. Stress following illness, if its severity exceeds that to be expected for the illness or if it is more severe than the environmental circumstances seem to justify, may be considered within the realm of abnormal illness behaviour. The evidence on abnormal illness behaviour and recovery has now accumulated to a point where it must be given the status of a contributory factor when considering the immediate and long term sequellae of almost all acute and chronic illness states.

Management of Stress After Illness

Stress management has received a great deal of attention in the psychological literature. While it is common to think that stress management defines a circumscribed set of procedures or techniques uniquely developed for and therefore solely suited to the management of stress disorders in individual patients, stress management in reality takes psychological procedures and therapeutic strategies from all areas of psychology and psychiatry. It is their end objective, the relief of stress and its symptoms, rather than the origins of the therapeutic procedures which gives stress management its name.

Five broad categories of psychological intervention strategies are typically drawn on to construct stress management packages or programs suited to individual patients. The most prominent among these is *relaxation training or therapy*. The establishment of the relaxation response by the use of muscle tension/relaxation exercises is well understood and widely regarded in stress management. It is based on a simple technology requiring no equipment and may be easily applied by nurses in the hospital ward setting. Muscle relaxation is clearly at odds with the peripheral symptoms of tension so characteristic of the stress response, and its establishment, therefore, acts as an effective counter to the unpleasant and often painful symptoms of this response. Its simplicity and ease of application, together with its ready acceptability by most patients, the almost immediate relief it frequently gives from symptoms of stress, the absence of side effects and its broad relevance to most states of psychological distress make relaxation therapy the initial procedure of choice in stress management. The main disadvantage of relaxation alone is that while it effectively counters symptoms of the stress reaction, it does not address the cause of that reaction, namely environmental stressors and their interpretation by the individual.

Thus, *cognitive psychotherapy* is often used in conjunction with relaxation in stress management programs. This psychological intervention is based on the well recognised notion in stress research that environmental situations precipitate stress reactions only when individual cognitive frameworks interpret them to be potentially threatening or challenging. Cognitive psychotherapy encourages the individual to examine interpretations of environmental events and to reassess their threat or challenge in the light of rational analysis of their content and meaning. In doing so, it attempts to replace stressful interpretations of the environment with more rationally based and hopefully less stressful ones, thus limiting the severity of the stress response. Clearly, the objective nature of some stressors, serious illness among them, will nearly always result in realistic stress of some kind; cognitive psychotherapy does not aim to replace a real world with an ideal one, but merely to allow the individual to respond objectively to environmental threat or challenge. Its main advantage is that it addresses the central issue of the stress response, that is, the way individuals interpret their own unique environments. It is not so simply based as relaxation therapy, and requires a trained therapist with skills in encouraging examination and reassessment of stressor interpretation. As such, it is typically restricted to patients in whom the stress response is severe or for whom relaxation therapy on its own is insufficient.

The management of specific biological symptoms of the stress response which are broadly responsive to relaxation may require more directly based procedures, and *biofeedback techniques* provide a possible set of strategies in this respect. The aim of biofeedback is to allow the individual to establish voluntary control over specific physiological responses to stressors, for example heart rate, blood pressure or muscle tension. The focus of this control is determined by the magnitude of the physiological response to stressor exposure and by the physiological modality which, by the severity of its arousal response, poses the greatest potential threat to physiological stability. Biofeedback, which involves the process of developing awareness of physiological arousal and alteration of that arousal, by small degrees, to baseline levels, requires time, patience and sophisticated equipment. However, as portable equipment is developed for use in ward situations by those practitioners not specifically trained in psychology, the potential use of this set of procedures may increase considerably.

Of course, stress management may rely wholly on traditional, *supportive psychotherapy* of the kind outlined in Chapter 2. In this case, the nurse may be called upon to supply nothing more than a supportive, empathic and caring psychotherapeutic relationship allowing the patient to share problems, work through anxiety and cope more easily, though in a general way, with stressors and their consequences.

Finally, *pharmacological therapy* has an important place in stress management. This involves the use of drugs to assist in the control of the stress reaction. Minor tranquillizers have traditionally been the drugs of choice in the pharmacological management of the stress reaction, though in recent times the use of beta blockers has assumed some prominence, particularly when excessive arousal of the autonomic nervous system poses a problem. As with relaxation therapy, the use of drugs merely controls the symptoms of the stress reaction and does nothing for the causes. Moreover, the potential side effects of long term drug therapy must be a consideration in stress management where the stress reaction is likely to be prolonged. However, as an immediate form of relief from physiological distress associated with the stress reaction, the use of psychotropic medication may prove both useful and effective.

Summary

In this chapter we have looked at theories and models of stress, and at some of the evidence linking stress with the onset of illness and with recovery from it. The importance of this area of psychology for the practice of nursing is self-evident. Much of what nurses see in their clinical activities will relate to stress; arguments regarding stress will figure strongly in the illnesses of the patients they are caring for, and stress reactions to these illnesses themselves will be evident in the nurses' day to day contact with their patients. Indeed, the need to manage such reactions, as we will discuss in the next chapter, will form an important part of nurses' activities. The psychology of stress, then, might be seen as one of the most central areas of consideration in the practice of nursing.

References/Reading List

Alexander, F. (1950). *Psychosomatic Medicine*. New York: Norton.

Brady, J.V. (1958). Ulcers in 'executive' monkeys. *Scientific American*, 199, 95–100.

Breuer, J. & Freud, S. (1895). *Studies on Hysteria*. London: Hogarth Press.

Brown, G. & Harris, T. (1978). *Social Origins of Depression: A Study of Psychiatric Disorder in Women*. New York: Free Press.

Byrne, D.G. & Rosenman, R.H. (eds) (1990). *Anxiety and the Heart*. New York: Hemisphere Publishing Corporation.

Cannon, W.B. (1915). *Bodily Changes in Pain, Hunger, Fear, and Rage*. New York: Appleton.

Dunbar, F.H. (1943). *Psychosomatic Diagnosis*. New York: Hoeber.

Friedman, H.S. & Dimatteo, M.R. (1989). *Health Psychology*. Englewood Cliffs, New Jersey: Prentice-Hall.

Friedman, M. & Rosenman, R.H. (1974). *Type A Behavior and Your Heart*. New York: Knopf.

Henderson, S., Byrne, D.G. & Duncan-Jones, P. (1981). *Neurosis and the Social Environment*. Sydney: Academic Press.

Holmes, T.S. & Rahe, R.H. (1967). The Social Readjustment Rating Scale. *Journal of Psychosomatic Research*, 11, 213–218.

Horowitz, M.J. (1976). *Stress Response Syndromes*. New York: Jason Aronson.

Hoyenga, K.B. & Hoyenga, K.T. (1984). *Motivational Explanations of Behavior: Evolutionary, Physiological, and Cognitive Ideas*. Monterey, California: Brooks/Cole.

Lachman, S.J. (1972). *Psychosomatic Disorders: A Behavioristic Interpretation*. New York: John Wiley & Sons.

Lazarus, R.S. (1966). *Psychological Stress and the Coping Process*. New York: McGraw-Hill.

Levi, L. (ed.) (1971). *Society, Stress and Disease*. Volume 1. London: Oxford University Press.

Martin, E.A. (ed.) (1987). *The Concise Medical Dictionary*. Oxford: Oxford University Press.

Miller, T.W. (ed.) (1989). *Stressful Life Events*. Madison, Connecticut: International Universities Press.

Reber, A.S. (1985). *Dictionary of Psychology.* Middlesex: Penguin.

Seyle, H. (1975). *The Stress of Life.* New York: McGraw-Hill.

Spielberger, C.D., Sarason, I.G., Strelau, J. & Brebner, J.M.T. (eds) (1991). *Stress and Anxiety.* New York: Hemisphere Publishing Corporation.

Weiss, R.S. (1973). *Loneliness: The Experience of Emotional and Social Isolation.* Cambridge, Massachusetts: MIT Press.

5
Emotions and the Helping Relationship

The Nature and Explanation of Emotions

Emotion, of one kind or another, is a ubiquitous accompaniment to illness, and one of the most widespread and enduring of all the attributes nurses will observe in their patients. The term 'emotion' has both a popular and a technical meaning. Popular usage ties emotion to an experiential response occurring when an individual encounters circumstances in the psychosocial environment requiring extremes of adaptation. The essence of emotion, however, is experiential; emotions are intense sensations within the individual, certainly coupled with attitudes, beliefs and perceptions regarding the surrounding environment and those in it. Above all, emotion is a state of felt sensation, the quality of which varies with the nature of the environmental precipitant.

Thus, in the simplest sense, emotions are synonymous with feelings, though the qualitative breadth of the former, the potential severity of their experience and the centrality of their existence to both theory and practice in psychology identify them as a unique field of study. Emotions are subjectively experienced states arising from quite specific environmental precursors. Anxiety, for example, is a state of extreme apprehension specifically linked to environmental circumstances of unpredictability coupled with threat. Depression is a state of profound grief closely associated with an environment from which there has been a loss of some important kind. But emotions are also the basis for the *motivation* of behaviours. An individual experiencing anxiety is quite distinctly motivated to seek a solution to the offensively uncertain environment while the depressed person may act to restore or replace the loss within his or her environment. Emotions are, therefore, not only inherently complex states of experience but also of fundamental importance to a complete understanding of human behaviour.

An old, but classically precise definition, provided by the theorist Magda Arnold in 1968, states that an emotion is: '. . . the felt tendency toward an object judged suitable, or away from an object judged unsuitable, reinforced by specific bodily changes according to the type of emotion' (p. 203). By a *felt tendency*, she meant the psychological attraction to or away from an object or situation depending, in some deciding way, upon the qualities of that situation, and by *judged suitable*, she meant the individual perception of the situation and the ensuing labelling of it which placed on it the construction of 'good' or 'bad'.

Arthur Reber, by contrast, in his *Dictionary of Psychology* (1985), decided that emotion was: '. . . utterly refractory to definitional efforts' (p. 235). Reber noted the origins of the term emotion to be with the Latin verb *emovere*, meaning to excite or to agitate. This, of course, implies more the motivational consequence of emotion than the common usage of the term as an experiential state. In this latter sense, Reber suggests emotion to be an umbrella term for an indistinct multitude of subjectively experienced states, the individual natures of which have no objective validity and are only really identified by the labels of depression, anxiety, love, anger and the like.

Regardless of how psychologists conceive of emotion, we typically share the view that it refers to a state of intensely felt experience, the various forms of which have common meanings for the large majority of people. The emotion of love, for example, while holding unique significance for those individuals experiencing it, and while bound both to the person (or object) evoking the emotion and the context in which it is evoked, none the less carries with it the universal meaning of extreme attraction to some external entity and a wish to direct unconditional nurturance towards that entity. This commonality of reference in the usage of specific emotional categories allows people to communicate easily deeply felt states or experiences, perhaps arising from similar environmental precipitants and within similar contexts, but certainly conveying messages of broadly shared meaning.

The accurate reception of these messages, and the initiation of appropriate responses to them, is a critical part of nursing practice. Patients across the whole spectrum of medical settings experience emotions specifically tied to their medical situations. While the subjective nature of the experience may be common to a wide variety of precipitants (the experience of anxiety, for example, is subjectively the same whether in response to the threat of a painful medical procedure or, say, the threat of a business failure), the capacity of the medical setting to evoke emotions is legion. Nurses, in the most routine of daily activities, will witness the full range of emotional responses among their patients, often at first in the form of intense anxiety and fear in response to threats to life, biological integrity and well-being, perhaps then transforming to strong anger or profound depression when the worst fears (real or imagined) are confirmed, or giving way to relief and joy when the threat to life or well-being is dismissed or removed.

Emotions, in the context of nursing practice, are present in a rich array of forms and intensities, unique in their implications for individual patients. They carry with them clear, universally understood meanings with equally clear expectations from patients of the responses they need (and sometimes demand) from nurses as they go about their tasks. People in trouble express their emotions not simply by a verbal message which is commonly understood ('I am *afraid*' or 'I feel *sad*') but also non-verbally, in their behaviours, the ways in which they respond to others, their capacity for rationality and decision making, and in their very willingness to continue existence in the world they see as the source of their troubles. Moreover, the experience and expression of emotions bear not only on the feeling state of the patient at any one point in time, but also on the progress of his or her illness and the speed and ease with which recovery and rehabilitation takes place. It is obvious, therefore, that this area is a mandatory one for understanding in any consideration of the psychological basis of the nurse's job.

A number of psychological and physiological theories have been put forward to explain the origins and appearance of emotions. These differ according to the emotion in question: theories of the origin of anxiety differ from those explaining anger, and these in turn, are different from theories directed towards depression, and so on. Several general theories have, however, been advanced to account for the appearance of undifferentiated distress in the face of an adverse or threatening psychosocial environment. An overview of some of these general theories illustrates a distinct and progressive shift away from theories relying on a biological/mechanistic interpretation of feelings and towards those emphasizing the dynamic interaction between the thinking, appraising individual and the complex, potentially threatening psychosocial environment.

James–Lange Theory

Though the theories of the psychologist William James and the physiologist C. G. Lange arose independently, they are so similar as to have been incorporated under the same umbrella. Essentially, they hold that when faced with a threat or challenge, all individuals respond with physiological arousal, initiated by and under the control of the autonomic nervous system. This arousal becomes manifest in elevations in the levels of many bodily or somatic functions, including heart rate, blood pressure, sweat gland activity, gastric secretion, muscle tension and so on (these have been discussed more fully in Chapter 4). Perception of these changes by the individual, once given verbal description and a label, then expressed as a complaint or a feeling of distress, becomes identified as emotion. The James–Lange theory accounts well for the perception of somatic disequilibrium now considered to be an integral component of emotion, but fails to explain wide variations in emotional experience (the experience, in other words, of specific emotions) or the different experientially based labels given to these and arising out of variations in environmental precipitants.

Cannon–Bard Theory

A variant of the James–Lange theory, the Cannon–Bard theory, largely attributable to the physiologist Walter Cannon, incorporated the idea that emotion derived its physiological character from *hypothalamic* control and its behavioural attributes from *cortical control*, with information regarding precipitants being relayed to both centres in the brain through the *thalamus*. While this theory is a little more sophisticated from a neuroanatomical perspective, it too fails to account for the experiential uniqueness of emotion.

Other Physiological Theories

As scientific method in neuroanatomy and neurophysiology allowed the description of pathways of neurological control in greater detail, theories of even greater biological sophistication arose. Of these, Papez' theory, which once more emphasized the dual roles of the hypothalamus in regulating the somatic component of emotion and the cortex in organizing the 'psychological' component, and McLean's theory, which proposed a central role for the *limbic system* of the frontal lobes, were prominent. Modern psychologists, however, have two major difficulties with these approaches. First, like all physiologically based theories, they fail to explain, or treat as incidental, the wide variability and separate experiential character of each of the several identified emotional states. Second, the strict neuroanatomical basis for their operation has not been confirmed by contemporary studies in neurohistology.

Behavioural Theory

While this held that all emotions were learned responses to environmental occurrences, which is not something most psychologists would want to dispute, it neither addressed the environmental origins of emotions nor the biological processes which underlay them. Behavioural theory does allow for the observed variation in emotional experience and expression, since it accepts that there can be infinite variation in learned associations. However, it ignores anything but the observable behaviour (which, of course, includes verbal and other expressions of intensely felt distress) and so does not consider the nature of the precipitating information or the complex processes which organize that behaviour into the observable responses important to the behaviourists.

Cognitive Appraisal Theory

The recognition that the experience of emotion, both qualitatively and quantitatively, is integrally linked to the nature of the precipitating environmental stimulus has given rise to the cognitive appraisal theory of emotion. In this theory, the experience of emotion, in its various forms, is seen as a collective psychological and physiological response which occurs only when an environmental stimulus which has been interpreted as impacting on the individual in some personally significant way is encountered. The essential feature of this theory is that it recognizes the importance played by some cognitive mechanism of environmental stimulus interpretation in evoking emotion: emotion is only experienced if particular constructions are placed on the incoming stimulus information from the environment. The interpretation of an environmental stimulus as threatening or challenging seems crucial to this process (we have discussed this in far greater detail in Chapter 4 which deals with the topic of stress). The major advantage of the cognitive appraisal theory is that it conveniently and cogently accounts for the wide individual variation so evident in the study of the emotions.

Types of Emotional Experience

It will be clear from what we have said above that emotions are experienced in a plethora of forms and intensities. Fear, love, hate, sadness, joy, aggression, surprise and disgust are all common and familiar to human experience. Simple existence makes the experience of some or all of these inevitable over the course of a lifetime. They may be experienced in the extreme or in moderation and the presence and nature of the environmental stimulus evoking the experience may be obvious, obscured by the context or, in some cases, unavailable to conscious recognition. But emotional experience is a common, perhaps everyday occurrence for the large majority of people. Indeed, the failure to experience and express an emotional response in the face of some environmental stimuli (personal threat or significant loss, for example) may be considered more abnormal, as we have seen in Chapter 1, than the expression of a time-limited emotional response of noticeable severity. However, some emotions are more important from a clinical perspective than others. They have been shown, in empirical studies, either to constitute states of illness themselves if they are severe and protracted, or to promote the development and exaggerate the duration of other illnesses in vulnerable individuals. Clearly, it is the recognition and understanding of these forms of emotional response which will be of greatest practical importance to the practice of nursing, and we will briefly discuss the nature and importance of three of these.

Anxiety

The experience of anxiety is seen and reported in most cultures and societies. This is cogently reflected in Rycroft's (1968) comment: 'Anxiety is such a common experience that one would be disinclined to believe anyone who claimed to be immune to it' (p. 1).

In many situations, and particularly those involving potential threat, it is, as we have said before, the expected response, and its absence under such circumstances would be considered abnormal. Perhaps the most comprehensive definition (description may be the more apt term) of anxiety was provided more than 30 years ago by Portnoy (1959) in the *American Handbook of Psychiatry*, when he wrote that anxiety was:

. . . subjectively experienced uneasiness, apprehension, anticipation of danger, doom, disintegration and going to pieces, the source of which is unknown to the individual and toward which he feels helpless, with a characteristic somatic pattern. This somatic pattern shows evidence of increased tension in the skeletal muscles (stiffness, tremors, weakness, unsteadiness of voice, etc.), the cardiovascular system (palpitations, blushing or pallor, faintness, rapid pulse, increased blood pressure etc.), and the gastrointestinal system (nausea, vomiting, diarrhoea etc.) (p. 123).

More recently, and somewhat more succinctly, Reber (1985) defined anxiety to be: '. . . a vague, unpleasant emotional state, with qualities of apprehension, dread, distress and uneasiness' (p. 43). Sarason & Sarason (1989) added to this broad view of anxiety, the experience, variously, of symptoms of: '. . . rapid heart rate, shortness of breath, diarrhoea, loss of appetite, fainting, dizziness, sweating, sleeplessness, frequent urination and tremors' (p. 145).

Broadly speaking, the criteria distinguishing normal from abnormal anxiety are that: (1) it should be more intense than the precipitating circumstances warrant, or should occur in the absence of apparent, external precipitants; (2) it should be more protracted than the precipitating circumstances explain; and (3) it should be beyond conscious, individual control. Even abnormal anxiety, however, is a relatively common experience; estimates vary but epidemiological studies have reported

that about 4% of the population experience clinical anxiety (of sufficient
severity to attract a psychiatric diagnosis), with a further 15% of the
population experiencing symptoms severe enough to impair personal
functioning, at any given time. In this light, it is clear that anxiety is not
a categorical state (present or not) but a continuous one, where the
intensity of the emotional distress may range from minor apprehension
to overwhelming and incapacitating panic.

One of the most important conceptual developments in the consideration of anxiety has been the view, put forward by the psychologist
Charles Spielberger, that it exists both as *state* and *trait*. This view, now
almost universally held by those investigating the origins and consequences of anxiety, distinguishes between an underlying and enduring
causal trait (a personality trait, in other words, and similar in some
respects to the notion of neuroticism) and periods or relatively temporary
states of manifest anxiety, evident in the form of subjectively experienced psychological distress accompanied by physical symptoms reflecting arousal of the autonomic nervous system. Trait anxiety, then,
may predispose an individual to state anxiety, the two being correlated
but open to independent psychometric measurement.

There are several fundamental features of anxiety. Though relatively
common, it is a distinctly unpleasant experience. It is an emotional state,
subjectively recognized as apprehension, fear or (most extremely) panic;
however, physiological arousal forms an integral component of its presentation, and elevations in cardiovascular function (heart rate, blood
pressure, relative blood distribution patterns, peripheral vasodilation),
gastrointestinal activity (gastric secretion, gut motility), skeletal muscle
tension and ecrine sweat gland activity are all commonly observed and,
in some cases, consciously perceived by those individuals in whom they
are occurring.

The presentation of anxiety and its impact on the individual will
constantly be observed in nursing practice. Anxiety may, in fact, be the
patient's primary complaint or symptom. This will be common in the
setting of the psychiatric hospital or outpatient centre, where the primary
anxiety disorders (i.e. psychological disorders involving overwhelming
anxiety as their predominant feature) are seen, diagnosed and treated.
There are mainly three relatively common anxiety disorders present at
this level. *Free-floating anxiety* or *anxiety neurosis* (severe anxiety
pervading the whole of the individual's conscious existence, but with no
apparent precipitant or cause in the external environment) poses a problem of substantial proportions because the absence of any explanatory
environmental cause makes it difficult both to understand and to treat.
Psychiatric explanations attributed its appearance to the presence of
unconscious conflicts in the individual personality, though these are
obviously not open to objective investigation, either clinically or in
research studies. Psychologists are therefore more inclined to look for
explanations in fears learned early in childhood, for which memories of

the original association have long since faded, leaving only the emotional response firmly evident but obscurely if at all connected to the present environment.

Phobic anxiety (anxiety or fear occurring only in the presence of a specific object or situation) is more straightforward. Phobic individuals will only experience and show anxiety when confronted with a feared object or situation, and at other times are free of the unpleasant emotional state. The anxiety response may, however, generalize from the primary phobic object or situation to others similar in form or nature. Thus, the person primarily phobic of spiders may generalize this to fear of all small, multi-legged creatures, and even to models or pictures of them. In extreme cases, phobic anxiety results in generalized behavioural avoidance, when the afflicted person avoids all situations in which there is a possibility of encountering the object that is feared. Such behaviour is clearly maladaptive and, on top of the extreme anxiety, is severely disruptive of everyday life. Psychologists find that the classical conditioning model of Pavlov provides a very useful explanation for the development of phobic anxiety, particularly where the connection between the feared object or situation and the experience of incapacitating anxiety defies rational understanding. While there is nothing inherently to be feared about cats, for example (a very young and naive infant shows no fear at all of cats or of any other animal), an adult phobic of cats may trace this back to the fortuitous pairing, usually in childhood, of consternation shown by another person (unconditioned stimulus) in the presence of a cat (conditioned stimulus) ultimately leading to fear (conditioned response) in the presence of cats. Just as learning theory provides a convincing explanation of the appearance of phobic anxiety, it also provides a framework for its elimination in the form of psychotherapy known as *behaviour therapy*.

Obsessive-compulsive disorder (characterized by extremes of ritualistic or avoidance behaviours) is the paradoxical member of the anxiety disorders since it does not involve the immediate presence of anxious emotion. Those people with obsessive-compulsive disorders, however, behave in ritualistic ways (rigidly patterned, highly organized behaviours including compulsive checking, invariantly structured modes of performing even the most simple daily tasks, overwhelming preoccupations with cleanliness and the like), only because not to do so would cause them to experience anxiety. The initiation of a ritualistic act or thought, or a compulsive behaviour, allows avoidance of anxiety. Once more, learning theory provides a compelling explanation for this form of anxiety disorder, this time in the form of operant conditioning. The avoidance of anxiety is strongly reinforcing and behaviours allowing this will become strengthened. Thus, the individual behaving in an apparently irrational, ritualistic way, will none the less persist in doing so because the behaviour serves to remove the anxiety which would otherwise be present. The initial appearance of anxiety is usually not able to be explained in obsessive-compulsive disorders, though some psychologists believe that it comes about through classically conditioned responses in childhood along much the same lines as the development of a phobia.

Nurses in the medical setting of a general hospital will also observe anxiety in their patients, but in this case as a contributor to, or as a secondary symptom in response to, the more primary presentation of physical illness. The physiological components of anxiety arising from autonomic hyperarousal may themselves assume the status of physical symptoms, stemming not so much from physical pathology as from intense emotional experience. In this situation, individuals may, because of genuine felt, physical distress, assume the presence of some physical illness (depending on the level of autonomic hyperarousal and the organ system it is mostly seen to engage), and come to identify themselves as 'patients' by seeking medical attention to alleviate their feelings of distress. This process, and the nurse's recognition of its presence and course, have clear implications for patient management.

Of course, there is now scientific evidence, as we have discussed more fully in Chapter 4, that the presence of severe anxiety, particularly if prolonged, may actually act upon the body's physiological functioning to cause tissue pathology and promote the onset of illness. The possibilities for intervention by nurses here are not quite so obvious since the influence of anxiety on health is seldom evident until health has been replaced by illness. Still, the role of nurses in the primary prevention of illness is becoming increasingly more prominent as medicine shifts from its preoccupation with the technical management of the patient after illness towards an equal concern with the modification of risk factors leading up to illness. In this respect, the early identification of anxiety by the nurse and its treatment either personally or by referral to a practitioner with appropriate psychological qualifications assume considerable importance.

Nurses will see anxiety most frequently, however, in the form of a response to an already established illness. Physical illness which is life threatening or which carries the probability of disability will produce the psychological response of anxiety. So too will illness which is painful or causes discomfort, or which involves painful or uncomfortable diagnostic or therapeutic procedures. Anxiety is a natural and expected response to any situation in which there is threat to survival or well-being. By extension, any situation which brings with it uncertainty or where outcomes are unsure or unpredictable has the potential to generate anxiety. Thus, even symptoms or physical sensations which have been demonstrated not to be life threatening may bring about anxiety if the individual is uncertain of their real meaning or significance for illness, or is unpersuaded of their innocuous nature by available medical (including nursing) opinion.

The nurse comes into almost daily contact with patients who, because of actual or imagined threat of or from illness, will manifest and express anxiety in many ways. For some patients it will be an open, unashamed cry for help and assurance. For others it will come in the more masked form of withdrawal, agitation or complaint. In ways we have suggested above, the physical components of anxiety can add to the symptoms already being suffered by the patient, and in doing so, both increase the overall level of distress and obscure the clinical picture relevant to the illness under treatment. There is also good evidence now that severe anxiety in response to many illnesses may act to delay recovery from those illnesses and increase the period of time necessary for rehabilitation. Autonomic arousal can create physiological conditions opposed to the reversal of many kinds of tissue pathology, while the psychological components of anxiety may lead to behaviours at odds with compliance with therapeutic regimes. Consider, for example, the patient recovering from myocardial infarction. Autonomic arousal, as part of anxiety, may liberate cardiologically dangerous levels of catecholamines (neurotransmitter substances) into the myocardium (the heart muscle) so challenging the heart at a biologically vulnerable time. At the same time, psychological anxiety regarding the possibility of recurrence may inhibit the patient from engaging in rehabilitative exercise. There are many examples like this which could be taken from daily nursing practice. It is essential, therefore, both to recognize reactive anxiety in patients recovering from illness, and if it is severe or inappropriate to arrange for anxiety management in a manner consistent with ongoing medical treatment.

The patient, however, is not the sole possessor of anxiety in the medical setting. Parents, husbands and wives, other family members and friends will all experience anxiety associated with the patient's illness. Uncertainty generates anxiety in these people too, and this may impose itself upon the nurse's role. If they are dependent on the patient, their anxiety may stem from uncertainty about their own future well-being. And anxiety may, in fact, be passed on from the patient to others; reciprocal anxiety is the phenomenon in which patient anxiety is matched, in nature and severity, by anxiety experienced by significant others. Indeed, nurses, too, may become anxious in the course of their caring role, either through concern for the outcomes of their patients or through uncertainty regarding the correctness and effectiveness of their own nursing care.

Anxiety is, then, the ubiquitous emotion. It is universal to nursing settings of all kinds and equally widespread among the whole range of patients that nurses will interact with during the course of their professional careers. Recognition of anxiety in the patient, in significant others and in themselves is an essential skill for nurses who are to be more than simple technicians.

Depression

Like anxiety, depression is a widespread form of affective distress, continuous in nature and experienced in one form or another by most individuals throughout the course of a lifetime. Depression was broadly defined in Reber's *Dictionary of Psychology* as: '. . . a mood state characterized by a sense of inadequacy, a feeling of despondency, a decrease in activity or reactivity, pessimism, sadness and related symptoms . . .' (p. 188). Somewhat more specifically, Aaron Beck (1967) wrote of depression that it was a psychopathological process defined by the attributes of:

(1) a specific alteration in mood: sadness, loneliness, apathy; (2) a negative self-concept associated with self-reproaches and self-blame; (3) regressive and self-punitive wishes: desires to escape, hide or die; (4) vegetative changes: anorexia, insomnia, loss of libido: and (5) change in activity level: retardation or agitation. (p. 7)

Under some circumstances, as we shall discuss later, depression is the normal, expected response to a range of life events having to do with loss. It shifts from normal to abnormal when it satisfies the same criteria distinguishing normal from abnormal anxiety (that is, when its severity and/or duration are disproportionately high relative to the nature of the precipitant). As a phenomenon of abnormal psychology, depression will be seen in a number of guises and contexts as nurses go about the daily care of their patients.

Depression may exist as a psychiatric entity in its own right, comprising not simply the emotional symptom of depression (profound grief or sadness are common synonyms) but accompanied by a set of associated symptoms both psychological and physiological in form, delineating a clinical condition of complex presentation. Indeed, the literature in abnormal psychology suggests that several diagnostic kinds of depression exist, all sharing the common thread of depressed mood but qualitatively different from one another in accompanying symptoms. The diagnosis of depression has proved a troublesome exercise in abnormal psychology, but there is general agreement on the view that as a psychiatric entity depression is not a unitary but a multi-state concept. There is less agreement on the particular combinations of accompanying symptoms identifying each of these clinical states and separating them from one another.

The most severe depression is to be found in that clinical state called *endogenous* or *psychotic depression*. Here, the individual is stricken with crippling sadness, usually accompanied by feelings of helplessness, hopelessness and imagined guilt, often involving loss of motivation and retardation of motor functions as well as loss of appetite (anorexia) and sleep disturbance, and all too often ending tragically in suicide or in attempts at it. Though the psychological origins of depression are usually seen as a response to the loss of a valued person, object or state of being, psychotic depression arises in the apparent absence of any such environmental precipitant. It is most often seen in middle age and in those with no previous history of psychiatric disorder. Current views of its cause tend towards biological explanations, and there is quite persuasive evidence that disturbed patterns of synthesis and utilization of catecholamines (neurotransmitter substances of which the most well recognized are adrenalin and noradrenalin) at particularly critical locations within the central nervous system are responsible for this condition. Not surprisingly, though psychological treatments are widely used, endogenous depression is often effectively managed with antidepressant medication.

Arguably less severe (on average) but certainly more common is *reactive* or *neurotic depression*. As the name suggests, this clinical state occurs in response to some identifiable environmental precipitant usually associated with the real, anticipated or imagined loss of some person, object or state of being. Loss of a close relative or friend through death or separation may precipitate reactive depression, as may loss of inanimate objects if they are sufficiently valued. Loss of a role or occupation (broadly, a state of being) may also precipitate reactive depression, because of not only the anticipated material loss this may bring but also the decrease in perceived self-worth which follows from such a life change. Reactive depression, like endogenous depression, is not just a symptom of sadness or grief but a clinical entity with accompanying symptoms of agitation, complaint, sleep disturbance and autonomic hyperarousal. In this latter respect, it resembles the symptoms of anxiety its other label of neurotic depression implies.

Given the importance of identified environmental loss in the cause of reactive depression, the role of the psychosocial environment has assumed some prominence in the search for explanations. A surfeit of life events (typically those involving loss or exit) in the absence of adequate social support (as we have discussed in Chapter 4) has been found in many studies of the genesis of reactive depression. Of recent interest, as well, is the theory that opportunities for social learning during early childhood may present the developing individual with experiences reinforcing the view that they have little or no control over the misfortunes of life. The ensuing conviction of helplessness in the face of life events becomes learned through repeated occurrences, and the individual grows up with *learned helplessness*, resulting in the experience of depression whenever a situation occurs which threatens challenge or possible misfortune. In the light of the considerable prevalence of reactive depression in modern societies, much research effort is presently being put into the investigation of causes, and a combination of psychosocial and learning theories currently occupies greatest attention. The patently psychological nature of reactive depression suggests that psychologically based therapies will be most effective in its treatment, and this is largely borne out by the available evidence.

A variant of reactive depression, and one which will occur more frequently in nursing practice, is that of depression simply as a symptomatic response to a more primary medical condition. Depression may certainly exist as an isolated emotional symptom, occurring in response to environmental stressors. Unlike true reactive depression, however, the primary manifestation is depressed mood alone, and the accompanying symptoms which might endow it with the status of an independent clinical entity are not, and need not be, present. Thus, deep depression may be seen in response to the diagnosis of a severe or life threatening illness, but as a secondary response to that illness and not as an independent clinical entity. The diagnosis of illness, particularly if severe, life threatening or protracted, has clear implications for potential loss. At the most obvious level, there may be loss of income due to a lost or reduced capacity to work. Illness may threaten the loss of relationships as it impairs the physical or interpersonal capacity to maintain these. It may bring about loss of lifestyles and social roles as it reduces the ability to function in occupational, family and recreational settings. As such, illness may threaten the loss of self-esteem and the potential for pleasure and enjoyment. Illness may, in fact, signify the loss of a self-image built up over years of development and experience; a woman who has undergone a mastectomy or hysterectomy may loose her whole sense of femininity and sexuality while a man who has suffered a severe myocardial infarction may find his masculine image of strong husband and able provider largely destroyed. Illness, then, is intimately bound up with the possibility of loss, and depression as a response to illness is completely understandable.

Primary and secondary depression are often confused, particularly within the context of a medical setting, and this may lead to errors of management which not only fail to alleviate the mood disturbance of a depressive reaction but may complicate the clinical presentation of the primary medical complaint. The accurate recognition of depression within the medical setting, in whatever form it takes, is therefore an important part of nursing practice. Common instruments for the measurement of depression typically include items to assess symptoms in the categories of (1) mood and suicidal intent, (2) ideation, beliefs and attitudes, (3) psychomotor speed and behaviour, and (4) somatic or psychophysiological distress. Nurses, familiar with these symptoms and with the distinction between depression as a clinical entity and depression as an emotional response to illness will be more closely attuned to the complete needs of their patients than those who see patient depression as just one more problem to be coped with in the technical process of keeping people alive.

Depression, like anxiety, varies widely in severity from one individual to another, from mild sadness and gloom to overwhelming despair. Estimates of the prevalence of clinical depression vary between studies and populations, but assessment of random samples of unselected populations suggest that around 2% of men and 4% of women will experience depression of clinical magnitude (that is, of a severity significantly impairing the capacity to live and function adaptively, and therefore requiring treatment) at any point in time. The prevalence of short term depression as an emotional response to illness is far higher, and studies have suggested that up to 20% of patients receiving outpatient treatment (or attending a general practitioner) and 50% of patients hospitalized for their illness will respond with depression at some time during the course of that illness.

One epidemiological feature of the rate of observed depression is the quite noticeable sex difference. Women report depression at undeniably higher frequencies, and of arguably higher magnitudes or severities, than do men. This is a well established phenomenon. Some epidemiologists and psychologists believe that this observed difference reflects reality; that is, for reasons not well understood but most likely related to a combination of biological and social vulnerabilities, women actually experience depression more often and more severely than men. Others have argued that the observation is an artefact of reporting; that is, because women have been socialized to express emotion more readily than men, they will report depression more often to their medical attendants and manifest it more clearly to those around them (by crying and so on) than will men. Men, by contrast, having been socialized (at least in Western cultures) to suppress emotional expression in case they are considered unmasculine, will admit to depression only with reluctance, but will report other symptoms (physical distress) or adopt other behaviours (anger and hostility or alcohol consumption) as so-called depressive equivalents.

The evidence surrounding this argument is far from clear. The sex difference seems as apparent in cultures where emotional expression is more openly allowed and observed in men. Moreover, examination of the symptoms making up clinical depression shows that sex differences are evident not just in reported mood but also in psychomotor and psychophysiological symptoms, where one would not really expect the operation of cultural or socialized constraints on reporting. Whatever the explanation, nurses will observe a greater rate of depressive responses to illness among their female patients than they will among males, and must be cautious not to assume that male patients not overtly showing distress in the face of illness are as totally free from depression as their external appearance would indicate.

Anger

Anger is the forbidden emotion in many societies because of its potential for violence and destruction. Yet, though it is frowned upon and discouraged, anger is evident, either overtly or covertly, in response to a multitude of situations. Reber (1985) defines anger as: '. . . a fairly strong emotional reaction which accompanies a variety of situations such as being physically restrained, being interfered with, having one's possessions removed, being attacked or threatened . . .' (p. 35).

The presence of anger may be identified by external signs of threat, for example facial grimaces or body postures suggesting violent action, and the emotion has the potential to follow, from this, to actual behaviours of attack. Thus, while the experience of anger is restricted to the angry individual, the expression of anger may overflow on to others, perhaps for the most part only in the form of sharp verbalizations, but occasionally as physical harm. It is in the expression of anger that the emotion has achieved its taboo status, though even the experience of anger is seen by some subgroups in society to be inconsistent with good manners and conduct.

Anger is commonly used synonymously with hostility and aggression, but psychologist have suggested that the concepts are different and should be treated as such. According to this view, anger is no more than an emotional state which occurs in response to environmental situations involving frustration or threat to personal control. Hostility, by contrast, is characterized by a complex set of attitudes and predisposing beliefs which may lead the individual, in times of frustration, towards destructive actions aimed at removing the source of the frustration, whether this is another individual, organization or object. If removal of the source is not possible the individual may engage in generally unstructured, destructive behaviour. There is also evidence that hostility in an individual contributes to a broadly paranoid interpretation of the world and a tendency to view it and those in it with malevolent intent. Hostility has been consistently associated with strong competitive urges and with a prominent need for achievement, so that it has come to be considered characteristic of some, notably upper level occupational groups engaged in commerce and business pursuits. Aggression is the collective set of behaviours which occur when an angry individual, perhaps made that way by underlying hostility, acts to materially remove the source of frustration from her or his environment. Such behaviours are typically destructive, often disruptive of social harmony and order, and potentially harmful to those who form the objects or foci of aggression.

Within this context, the state/trait distinction, already applied by Spielberger to the emotion of anxiety, may be seen to apply equally to anger. The individual possessing a hostile personality (trait) and thus viewing the world with suspicion and malevolence, will more readily respond with anger (state) when that world presents frustrations than another, less hostile individual, who may see these same frustrations as mere inconveniences.

Perhaps because anger is the taboo emotion, and because it does not figure in the schema of psychiatric classifications as an identified clinical state, data on the prevalence of anger are singularly lacking in the psychological literature. Aggression, or the expression of anger in word or action, figures in the psychiatric formulations of a number of abnormal states. It is a clinical feature of the personality disorders where, poorly restrained by low impulse control, aggression may lead the individual to encounter difficulties with the law. Aggression has also been implicated in the genesis of depressive illnesses, though as an inward directed, and therefore suppressed condition rather than an overt state of behaviour aimed destructively at other individuals. Moreover, the trait variable of hostility has been suggested in a multitude of theories and speculations on the origins of psychological disorders to underlie a variety of psychopathological conditions, once more including depressive illnesses, but extending to such things as response to intractable pain. Scrutiny of the most up to date system of psychiatric classification, the *Diagnostic and Statistical Manual of the American Psychiatric Association*, third edition — revised (DSM III-R), however, shows that neither anger nor aggression constitute states of abnormal behaviour in their own right. They may contribute to the symptom patterns of other, more circumscribed disorders, or they may be included in the aetiological formulations of other conditions, but they do not attract diagnoses in isolation.

None the less, anger and its expression are part of normal, everyday life. Though it may not be socially condoned, anger is expected whenever there is a threat to personal control and dominance of individual environments. Whenever situations go in directions unplanned or unwanted by the individual, there is a potential for the response of anger to ensue. This is most often seen only as an emotional state, a felt reaction involving surging physiological arousal in the face of frustration. Occasionally, it may become manifest as action, sudden and intense, having the potential for violence and destruction but mostly confined to verbal outburst or harmlessly directed physical expression. More rarely, it may take the form of destructive action, seeking by force to remove the source of the frustration in a planned act of harm, or lashing out in an unstructured and uncontrolled way, directing aggression not so much at those individuals or objects responsible for the frustration, as at those most readily available at the time of the outburst. It is when anger and its expression in aggression becomes destructive and dislodged from personal control that it leaves normality and enters the realm of the pathological.

Nurses, then, will see anger as a symptom of psychological disorder within the setting of the psychiatric hospital or outpatient clinic. However, because of the capacity of physical illness to threaten personal integrity, frustrate long-planned and valued activities, and remove control of life from the individual to the technical but largely impersonal skills of others, nurses will most often see anger as a response to illness in patients they care for within the strictly medical setting. Anger is an established and accepted stage in the process of psychological adaptation to illness in which there is a threat or a certainty of death. Having first experienced grief and depression, people facing death will revolt angrily against objects and people in the environment seen (correctly or otherwise) to bear some responsibility for the threat, and perhaps even against the perceived unfairness of the world for having thrust this upon them. There is often no rationality guiding the direction of such anger, though observational research strongly suggests that it is a necessary phase to negotiate if the dying person is to resolve his or her fear of death and come to accept its inevitabilty with calmness. Nurses working in the care of the terminally ill, or in those areas of nursing where life threatening illness is managed, will see this anger daily. They will also see anger, of a similar magnitude and sequence, in those close to the patient. Close relatives and friends will respond with anger, sometimes strongly, at the frustration of lost control over the lives of the people they love.

Anger will be expressed, both by patients and by those close to them, at a system seen to be responsible for the failure of medical treatment to prolong life or restore physical integrity, the imposition of lengthy and painful treatments, the restriction of free movement and action which sometimes necessarily accompanies the medical management of serious illness or injury, and the seeming incapacity of many medical practitioners to explain what is wrong, what they are doing by way of diagnosis and treatment, and why this is being done. It is nurses who are most often the primary focus of this anger, not because they are responsible, but because they are there.

The young man, angry at his immobilization in an orthopaedic ward following a vehicle accident, the mother, angry that her child is in pain after surgery, the middle-aged man, angry that he should suffer a heart attack just prior to a busy period in his business, will all project that anger onto nurses, because it is nurses who are most frequently seen and identified with the system. Others in the medical team can enter at specified times, perform their diagnostic or treatment functions, and disappear to the anonymity of the laboratory or the consulting room, but nurses must constantly care for their patients. They are always within range. The observation of anger, and the need to deal with it in constructive and caring ways, are common to nursing practice. The need for self-protection in the face of anger, which is after all the emotion most closely associated with harm and destruction, is essential for the nurse's survival.

Denial

There are times, for the large majority of individuals, when the personal significance of the environmental threat is so great as to overwhelm them. Under these circumstances, some individuals may choose (consciously or otherwise) to disregard completely the existence of the threat or to ignore its objective significance, interpreting the situation instead as posing a threat of relatively low personal significance. As a result, the intense emotional response which might have been expected is circumvented or reduced to a response of a lesser, more personally comfortable intensity. When this happens, the individual is said to be *denying* or to be using the mechanism of *denial*.

In the terminology of Freud, denial is a *defence mechanism* or a mode of information processing designed to protect the individual against distress arising from awareness of threatening elements in the environment. Denial achieves this by disregarding those elements or by reinterpreting them in less threatening ways. As the psychoanalytic theorist Norman Cameron (1963) has said: '. . . adults deny what they perceive, think or feel in a traumatic situation, either by saying something to the effect that it can not be so, or else trying to invalidate something intolerable by deliberately ignoring its existence.' (p. 29).

Within the psychoanalytic context, denial is a completely unconscious 'act', set in place by response tendencies originating in the early years of a child's development. In the adult, the mechanism is brought into play whenever a potential threat is encountered, and acts as an effective, if somewhat short term, protection against distress.

One does not, of course, need to accept the unconscious nature and operation of denial, or even its psychoanalytic origins, to observe that it exists. The view that denial may be a mechanism of conscious choice, but still designed to achieve the purpose of protection against the distressing qualities of a threatening environment, does not at all invalidate its observed existence. Indeed, some individuals may openly state that they are able to cope with a threatening environment, and avoid undue distress, by consciously choosing not to think about the threat or by deliberately construing the environment in ways less threatening.

Denial will be observed, within the nursing context, in a plethora of forms and situations. Generally, illness poses a threat to the survival or to the integrity of the individual, and as we have discussed above episodes of illness are typically responded to with emotional distress in one form or another. The intensity of this distress will be a function of the objective severity of the illness and the threat to life or future performance that it poses (a heart attack or cancer will pose a greater objective threat than, say, appendicitis or influenza). The intensity will also be determined by those attributes of the individual personality which underlie self-image and regulate coping behaviours (a person whose self-esteem revolves largely around sporting activities and physical prowess will experience greater distress in response to an illness limiting physical exercise and mobility than will someone whose self-image is fixed to more intellectual pursuits). Thus, the operation of denial and the readiness with which it is brought into use (consciously or otherwise) in threatening situations will depend not just on the objectively assessed severity of a given illness and on the anticipated degree of distress which might arise from it, but also on the unique and personally specific threat which that illness poses to the self-image of any individual.

In the short term, denial may be quite adaptive both medically and behaviourally. The patient using moderate degrees of denial in response to illness may be less complaining and demanding, more compliant with non-medical requests and intent on presenting an image of normality. Denial may, however, also lead to angry confrontations, when the nurse, charged with the administration of medical care, must undertake activities in conflict with the patient's unreal view of the severity of their illness. This may take the form of conflict when the patient's rejection of illness and of its implications is at odds with compliance with medical instructions or with submission to medical procedures necessary for the management of the illness. In extreme forms, denial may result in premature discharge by the patient from hospital care. For most patients, denial simply results in a reinterpretation of the meaning of illness so as to decrease the degree of experienced emotional distress. For some, however, total denial may be the only way they see of coping, and so they will tell themselves and everyone around them that the illness does not exist, using rationalizations of mistaken diagnosis, unreliability or errors in test results, mistaken identities of test results incorrectly labelled or named, and even the incompetence of staff, including nursing staff, as a means of reinforcing this belief.

Denial, then, has clear implications for a return to health after illness, and the recognition of this state by the nurse is of equally clear importance. The absence of emotional responses to undeniably serious illness or the blunting of emotions under the same circumstances provides good evidence of denial in operation. While it is conceivable that the patient is simply the fortunate possessor of an accepting, stoic approach to misfortune, the bulk of evidence on emotions and their environmental precipitants makes it far more likely that denial is masking a more normal and expected emotional state, not consciously experienced at the time but dormantly awaiting expression. Broad failure to comply with medical and nursing care is also an indication of denial. So too is a stance in which the patient continually disputes the need for care and the form it takes. And in the extreme, as we have said, denial may even lead the person to deny completely the presence of illness and to refuse to become a patient, resulting, in turn, in the blanket refusal of treatment.

In discussing the recognition of denial, one word of caution is necessary. Patients have undeniable rights to question those who provide medical care for them, to request disclosure of the fullest possible information on their illness and its treatment, and to dispute what seems to them to be lacking in sense and justification. The rational application of these rights should not be taken as an indication of denial, and the 'diagnosis' of denial should never be used as an excuse for disregarding the patient's psychological needs during the course of nursing care. The recognition that a patient is denying the real impact of illness may, however, result in the use of simple counselling aimed at breaking down denial, allowing the ownership of important emotions to emerge, and (as we will discuss later) perhaps facilitating the process of recovery from illness or rational acceptance of its inevitable consequences when recovery is not possible.

Determinants of the Emotional Response

Several of the general factors determining the probability and magnitude of emotional responses in the face of environmental threat, particularly from illness, have been discussed above. The actual or objective severity of the illness is clearly important, though, as we have seen, the ways in which the individual perceives the illness and interprets its personal significance have an equal if not greater influence on the appearance and extent of the emotional response. Thus, in considering the origins of the various emotions, we must look both at the precipitating characteristics of the environment and at the individual's personal constructions of that environment.

The complexity of the psychosocial environment ensures an abundance of potential stressors or precipitants which have the capacity to evoke emotional responses of various kinds. Even within the more restraining context of illness, there is the potential for the precipitation of a range of emotional responses of substantial breadth.

As we have discussed above, illness may bring with it uncertainty and unpredictability regarding outcomes. Most individuals who become ill have little or no information about their own biological functioning or what happens when illness disrupts this. The medical system is notorious for failing to redress this situation with the provision of clear, simple and freely given information throughout the course of the illness. It is one of the simplest rules of psychology that uncertainty generates anxiety. Indeed, there is evidence to suggest that certainty, even about the most unpleasant events, generates less anxiety than not knowing; people appear less anxious when they know they are going to die than when they fear they will die but do not know for certain. In this situation, the uncertainty resulting from the (more often than not) failure of the 'system' to provide information indicates anxiety as an almost inevitable response to illness. Even when the patient has access to all necessary information provided in language or in other ways that they understand, unpredictability about the future may still be there. The patient may be uncertain about the chances of recurrent illness, the capacity for financial survival or for future employment may be in doubt, the stability and viability of present relationships may be unpredictable in the future in the face of continued disability, and so on. Uncertainty and unpredictability may never be totally removed but the provision of information by the nurse who answers questions and offers factual reassurance in language capable of being understood by her patients will go far to achieving this.

Even if the present course of illness is more or less certain, and the future is reasonably predictable, the illness may then transform the patient's environment to one heralding either immediate or fore-shadowed loss, and grief or depression may closely follow. Illness, as we have seen earlier in this chapter, can result in both tangible and intangible losses. Loss of self-esteem or self-image is no less real than material loss or loss of physical integrity, and the consequences of each may be indistinguishable from one another. While uncertainty can be counteracted by the provision of information, loss arising from illness or its effects is more resistant to direct intervention.

It is not within nurses' power to restore the patient's real or antici-pated material loss arising from illness. Neither are nurses able, when illness involves permanent or extended physical incapacity, to restore immediately or conveniently the patient's physical or biological integ-rity. Loss of self-esteem or self-image may be open to intervention by the use of counselling methods discussed in Chapters 2 and 3, but even this is likely to require a concentrated and extended effort either beyond the psychotherapeutic capabilities of clinical nurses (and requiring refer-ral to a clinical psychologist), or greater than the time commitment they are able to make to a single patient. Once more, then, listening in a sensitive way and the capacity to identify patients with situations of loss requiring specialist intervention must be within nurses' routine set of clinical skills.

Illness undoubtedly removes control of life from the individual to others more concerned with technical rather than interpersonal skills, and this carries with it frustration and resultant anger. As we have also shown, then, anger is another common and expected emotional response to an environment in which illness is a prominent characteristic. Nurses, of course, are part of the system responsible for the removal of control and may be seen by the patient as the source of frustration. Since they are most often in direct contact with the patient, it is they who may become the principal focus for the expression of anger. As with loss, nurses may have little capacity to restore control to the patient and remove the sources of frustration. Their actions will be constrained by their role and by the system within which it occurs. Empathic understanding of the patient's situation, of the loss of control dominating it, and of the in-evitable anger which this precipitates may be their only tool in dealing with this problem. They will need to acquire the ability to communicate that understanding back to the patient, and for themselves the recog-nition that the anger is system generated rather than directed at them personally will be an essential point for nurses to remember.

As we have seen, then, when a person becomes ill and assumes the role of a patient, that person's environment takes on a new capacity to precipitate emotions. Moreover, it is the clinically significant emotions of anxiety, depression and anger which are most often seen in response to illness. We must look, however, not just at the nature of the precipitating environment but also at the characteristics of the individual to gain the most complete understanding of emotional responses to illness. In Chapter 4, we discussed individual determinants of the stress response within the context of influences on the interpretive process, and in a general sense, the factors discussed there bear directly on the determination of emotions. However, there are several additional individual factors which must be considered when looking at the emotional response to illness.

Foremost among these is past experience with illness. Just as past experience with stressors in general influences the ways in which people will respond to the same stressors in the future, so experience of past episodes of a particular illness will bear strongly on emotional responses to future episodes of the same illness. Broadly speaking, past experience of an illness is expected to reduce the intensity of emotional responses to some future episode, since there is greater certainty and predictability regarding the course of the illness and its expected outcome. Evidence suggests that the victim of a second heart attack, for example, obviously aware of the fact that a heart attack is eminently survivable, is less emotionally affected than when it occurred the first time. Where recurrent illness promises severe pain or discomfort, however, or where recurrence strongly increases the chance of death or significant disability, the emotional response can well be accentuated by a quite different set of expectations.

The personal social context within which illness occurs will also influence the emotional outcome. An individual in socially stable, financially secure circumstances, for example, will typically respond with less emotional intensity to an illness threatening loss of working capacity than will a socially and interpersonally isolated individual in need of work to survive. The evidence on emotional responses to illness documents a host of socioeconomic associations, but it is clear that those from poorer socioeconomic backgrounds respond more adversely than those who are better off. While this certainly relates to matters of social and financial security, it may also relate to education and to an individual's capacity to understand the nature and consequences of their illness and the information given to them by medical staff, including nurses.

In practical terms, what this simply means is that all individuals are unique and that their emotional responses to illness, inevitable as they are, will be shaped and determined by the particular characteristics of the individual. No two sets of determining characteristics will be the same, and it cannot be assumed that simply because the illness is identical all sufferers of that illness will display the same intensity or quality of emotional response. Nurses must recognize the uniqueness of the individual condition and the highly specific influence this will have on emotional responses to illness. Acceptance of this in clinical practice will enable medical staff to avoid categorizing or stereotyping which provokes resent and anger in patients.

Emotional Determinants of Outcome after Illness

As acute phenomena, emotional responses to illness present management challenges in their own right. Patients responding to episodes of illness with displays of excessive emotion will almost always be more difficult to nurse than those responding less extremely. At best, intense emotional responses to illness among patients will evoke reciprocal and negative emotions in nurses, leading to the potential for dismissal of significant symptoms as mere complaint, and avoidance, so far as is possible, of those patients exhibiting such responses. The short term consequences of this are obvious: nurses will become frustrated and vulnerable to burnout (as we shall see in Chapter 9) and patients will experience rejection, avoidance and there will be the distinct chance of neglect. Nurses' sensitivity to the inevitability of intense emotional responses in at least some of their patients, and their recognition that these responses are often beyond the conscious control of the patients, will help to circumvent this widespread problem.

There is now good evidence, however, to suggest that intense emotional responses to illness exert powerful influences on the psychobiological processes of recovery from and rehabilitation after illness. A growing number of both clinical and epidemiological studies are available to document the broadly deleterious effects of intense emotional response on illness outcomes. These potential effects may be divided into two kinds. First, the experience of acute distress in response to illness may promote behaviours at odds with recovery and return to health. Take, for example, the elderly woman who is so afraid after hip replacement surgery of the possibility that she will have even less mobility and more pain than before that she is reluctant to leave her hospital bed and the care it implies for her, and attempt her first steps towards independence; her emotional response of fear or anxiety leads her into a pattern of behaviour opposed to recovery and rehabilitation. Consider, alternatively, the young man who is so angry at the connotation of weakness and frailty his diagnosis of diabetes mellitus carries with it, that he rebels against dietary control of any kind; his emotional response, too, promotes a pattern of behaviour inconsistent with health. A similar situation may be observed for the operation of denial, where individuals refusing to accept the presence of illness or the demands it places upon them adopt or fail to alter behaviours at odds with recovery. The middle-aged, hitherto aggressively healthy man, faced with the diagnosis of angina pectoris, steadfastly denies that anything whatsoever could be wrong with his heart, and refuses to comply with advice to relax, reduce his weight, stop smoking and take more exercise. His refusal to change health-risk behaviours, because he denies the presence of the illness requiring this, places him at even greater risk of even more serious illness.

Second, intense emotional responses to illness may exert physiological effects which render the individual more vulnerable to complications of the present illness or more at risk of recurrent episodes of that illness. As we have discussed earlier in this chapter, and in more detail in Chapter 4, the process and experience of emotions have distinct physiological consequences. These are largely to be seen in elevations of activity within the autonomic nervous system and the neuroendocrine mechanisms regulating a great deal of bodily functioning. Emotions, for example, are closely associated with adrenal gland secretion of catecholamines which then circulate freely within the bloodstream and have an impact on all organ systems within the body. Organ systems physiologically unstable during the course of illness may easily be harmed by the complex and multi-focused stimulatory effects of autonomic excitation. Clinical evidence has now shown, for example, that the heart muscle (myocardium), the electrochemical regulation of which is highly physiologically unstable in the days following acute myocardial infarction, can quickly go into a potentially fatal arrhythmia in response to acute emotional distress.

Emotional responses, therefore, particularly if they are intense and prolonged, may seriously impede the processes of recovery and rehabilitation after many if not all illnesses. These responses have been discussed under the heading of *abnormal illness behaviour* in Chapter 4. It does not matter, in this situation, that the emotional response may be entirely consistent with the seriousness and threat of death imposed by the illness. Indeed, the most serious illnesses, and certainly those in which an intense emotional response is expected, may be the very illnesses least able to withstand the impact of extreme emotion. Two examples, those of coronary heart disease and cancer, may serve to illustrate these points more concretely.

Coronary Heart Disease

This regrettably common but undeniably serious illness carries with it the twin threats of death and protracted disability. Not surprisingly, clinical episodes of coronary heart disease are accompanied or immediately followed by emotional distress in the large majority of victims. These emotional responses typically take the form of anxiety in the short term. This steadily increases after onset of symptoms (chest pain, breathlessness and the like) and may become extreme on admission to hospital and to a coronary care unit, with the patient's realization that he or she is in the midst of a process which might end in death. Anxiety often subsides within a day or so of admission, when pain subsides, the patient feels more comfortable and recognizes that survival is probable. The setting of the coronary care unit brings with it the mixed feelings of security and fear; security because the patient knows that the best medical attention is on hand should complications arise, and fear because the patient also realizes he or she would not be there if they were not seriously at risk of death. The feeling of security usually overrides fear, however, as the patient spends time in the coronary care unit and survival becomes more and more certain; and in fact anxiety may return with considerable intensity around the time of discharge from the coronary care unit to the less highly monitored environment of the general medical ward. Anxiety can and does change to depression if it is not quickly resolved. Moreover, the threat to mobility and independence posed by coronary heart disease, and the strongly indicated need for lifestyle change in many patients, both have the capacity to evoke overt anger in these individuals. The whole range of possibly destructive emotions are, therefore, likely to be seen in response to coronary heart disease, and these have been documented in a good many clinical and epidemiological studies.

Part of this evidence has involved the prospective examination, over time, of the influence of emotional responses on outcome after clinical episodes of coronary heart disease, and it is now known that severe and prolonged emotional response to illness can lead to a range of unfavourable outcomes. In the short term, an intense emotional response to coronary heart disease can predispose to complications during hospitalization, including the occurrence of dangerous arrhthymias and even recurrent (and often fatal) infarctions. Patients showing such emotional responses tend to stay longer in coronary care units and longer in hospital; they place a greater demand on service delivery, including that of nursing, and are least able to be convinced of the ultimate survivability of a heart attack.

In the longer term, after discharge from hospital, patients experiencing intense emotional distress after coronary heart disease tend to return to work less speedily, to resume leisure pursuits and interpersonal contacts more reluctantly, and show a greater rate of psychological and social (including marital) pathology than patients showing more rational emotional responses to their illness. Very long term studies have also shown that extreme emotional response, particularly if it does not dissipate quite rapidly with recovery, is associated with recurrent and sometimes fatal episodes of coronary heart disease in the future.

Emotional responses to coronary heart disease have, therefore, been found to impair short term recovery and rehabilitation, impede return to work and social activities, and promote long term coronary morbidity and mortality. Not surprisingly, a great deal of current research in psychology is focusing on ways of limiting, managing and modifying intense emotional response in the face of coronary heart disease.

Cancer

The set of diseases, rightly or otherwise known by the collective label of cancer, also presents a far too common and frightening challenge in most countries of the world. Wherever the bodily location, the growth of a tumour or neoplasm will evoke a response, in the victim, of intense emotional distress. This is particularly to be seen where the tumour is confirmed as malignant, but strong emotional responses to non-malignant growths will also be observed, probably as a function of disbelief regarding the certainty of the diagnosis or a concern (largely false) that non-malignant tumours inevitably turn into malignant ones. Studies documenting emotional responses to a diagnosis of cancer suggest that, like coronary heart disease, the nature of the emotional response relates to the stage of the illness. Anxiety is common immediately on detection of symptoms (a lump in the breast, rectal bleeding or the like) and steadily progresses in intensity through the various diagnostic processes, often assuming clinical proportions if these processes are prolonged, indecisive or painful. Confirmation of the presence of malignancy is associated with the onset of depression, though this may coexist with anxiety. The patient often experiences hope as the course of treatment is planned and discussed, and the early stages of treatment, themselves typically heralding at least a short term disappearance of clinical signs and symptoms, are frequently associated with euphoria. Unfortunately, this is too often replaced with a return to distress when symptoms recur and a less favourable prognosis is pronounced. In terminal cases, many patients may achieve a state of calm acceptance, though this is typically not seen until other emotional states are resolved.

The most striking evidence for an influence of emotional responses on outcomes in cancer comes from work with victims of breast cancer. It has been found that patients who adopt and maintain an angry stance, vowing to beat the disease and return to a normal, healthy lifestyle, have far longer survival times than those who give up and resign themselves to what they see as the inevitable mortality of cancer. In this case, the presence of a so-called 'destructive' emotion, that of anger, seems actually to predispose to a favourable outcome, and though the patient may be difficult to deal with during this phase, the evidence clearly supports the value of the emotion. There is insufficient evidence to generalize this finding to survival from other forms of cancer. Moreover, the evidence conflicts with some scientifically less well founded but persuasively consistent reports that a state of calmness achieved through techniques of meditation may have beneficial effects on the survival chances of cancer sufferers.

The field of cancer is biologically complex, and the evidence on psychological contributions to its cause or course is as yet too inconclusive to allow broad generalizations. There is, however, good evidence that the emotions of anxiety and depression, at least, suppress key activities within the human immune system. In the light of extensive work implicating disturbances of immunity in both the cause and course of many cancers, however, there is good reason to continue to investigate the role of emotional responses in outcomes after a diagnosis of cancer.

Summary

This chapter explored the nature and explanations of emotions and demonstrated the relevance of emotional states to the practice of nursing. The chapter began by exploring the definition of emotions and enumerated a number of general theories which have attempted to explain the origins and appearance of emotional states. Four types of emotional experience were then considered, namely, the experience of anxiety, depression, anger and denial. It was shown that each of these emotional experiences have special relevance to patients recovering from illness. Determinants of emotional responses were also examined. Finally, the management challenges of handling patients displaying intense emotional responses to their illnesses, particulary patients suffering from coronary heart disease and cancer, were exemplified.

References/Reading List

Arnold, M.B. (ed.) (1968). *The Nature of Emotion*. Middlesex: Penguin.
Beck, A.T. (1967). *Depression: Clinical, Experimental and Theoretical Aspects*. New York: Hoeber.
Beck, A.T. & Emery, G. (1985). *Anxiety Disorders and Phobias: A Cognitive Perspective*. New York: Basic Books.
Brown, G. & Harris, T. (1978). *Social Origins of Depression: A Study of Psychiatric Disorder in Women*. New York: Free Press.
Byrne, D.G. & Rosenman, R.H. (eds) (1990). *Anxiety and the Heart*. New York: Hemisphere Publishing Corporation.
Cameron, N. (1963). *Personality Development and Psychpathology: A Dynamic Approach*. Boston: Houghton Mifflin.
Carson, R.C., Butcher, J.N. & Coleman, J.C. (1988). *Abnormal Psychology and Modern Life*. Glenview, Illinois: Scott, Foresman & Company.
Chesney, M.A. & Rosenman, R.H. (eds) (1985). *Anger and Hostility in Cardiovascular and Behavioral Disorders*. Washington: Hemisphere Publishing Company.
Karasu, T.B. & Steinmuller, R.I. (eds) (1978). *Psychotherapeutics in Medicine*. New York: Grune & Stratton.
King, N.J. & Remenyi, A. (eds) (1986). *Health Care: A Behavioural Approach*. Sydney: Grune & Stratton.

Levi, L. (ed.) (1977). *Emotions: Their Parameters and Measurement*. New York: Raven Press.

Levy, L.H. (1985). *Behavior and Cancer: Life-style and Psychosocial Factors in Initiation and Progression of Cancer*. San Francisco: Jossey-Bass Publishers.

Lipowski, Z.P. (1986a). Psychosomatic medicine: past and present. Part I. Historical background. *Canadian Journal of Psychiatry*, 31, 2–7.

Lipowski, Z.P. (1986b). Psychosomatic medicine: past and present. Part II. Current state. *Canadian Journal of Psychiatry*, 31, 8–13.

Lipowski, Z.P. (1986c). Psychosomatic medicine: past and present. Part III. Current research. *Canadian Journal of Psychiatry*, 31, 14–21.

Mandler, G. (1984). *Mind and Body*. New York: Norton.

Novaco, R.W. (1975). *Anger Control*. Lexington, Massachusetts: Lexington Books.

Portnoy, I. (1959). The anxiety states. In S. Ariete (ed.), *American Handbook of Psychiatry*. New York: Basic Books.

Reber, A.S. (1985). *Dictionary of Psychology*. Middlesex: Penguin.

Rycroft, C. (1968). *Anxiety and Neurosis*. London: Penguin.

Sarason, I.G. & Sarason, B.R. (1989). *Abnormal Psychology*. Englewood Cliffs, New Jersey: Prentice-Hall.

Scott, J., Williams, J.M.G. & Beck, A.T. (eds) (1989). *Cognitive Therapy in Clinical Practice: An Illustrative Casebook*. London: Routledge.

Spielberger, C.D. (1979). *Understanding Stress and Anxiety*. London: Harper & Row.

6
Communication in the Helping Relationship

Communication is central to all helping relationships since, without communication, the provider of help will be unable to convey to the recipient either the intent to help or the form in which help will be given. In nursing, where helping is paramount to success, communication occurs at many levels and in many contexts. Communication is affected by the individual's own attributes and by the settings or environments in which communication occurs. This chapter begins by exploring definitions and models which psychologists have put forward to explain the process of communication. In it, the focus is placed on communication as an interpersonal process, that is, a process in which the transfer of information takes place within a context of personal interaction. The functions of language and of verbal and non-verbal aspects of communications are all seen as part of the same system. In addition, barriers to effective communication between individuals and techniques for improving these communication skills will be detailed. Specific examples will be given to illustrate the importance of communication to the successful practice of nursing.

People communicate in unique and powerful ways, sharing broad forms but varying in the ways in which these forms are preferred and used. Communication is fundamental to most social processes. The expression of the most fundamental feelings by one individual to another, and the recognition by the recipient that such feelings have been expressed, requires the capacity to communicate effectively. Expressions of the most positive feelings of friendship, affection and love depend on an individual's ability to communicate these feelings in a language or form to which another individual will be receptive; so do expressions of the more negative feelings of anger, mistrust and hatred. In the practice of nursing, the capacity of nurses to communicate effectively to their patients that they are there to help, to care, to relieve pain and suffering or simply to understand that these exist is crucial to the effectiveness of the nurses' role.

In a broader perspective, communication is the dominant process of any organization (Smither, 1988) and failure of communication may easily undermine the efficient operation of that organization, clearly with potentially disastrous consequences where the lives of patients in situations of medical need are involved. When problems arise in organizations, no matter how these manifest themselves, their cause is frequently traced back to disruptions to or outright failures of communication (Schermerhorn, Hunt & Osborn, 1985). The continuing viability of organizations rests with the integrity of communication systems, and these in turn depend for their efficiency on the capacity of their elements, namely individual people, to receive, process and transmit information, one to another, in ways which maintain or enhance the meaning of that information, and add to the knowledge base or the sense of well-being of those to whom that information is ultimately passed on.

Defining Communication

Defining communication is no easy task. Communication is perhaps best seen as an interaction in which two or more people both send and receive messages, and in the process, both present aspects of themselves and interpret the presentations of others. We would probably all accept that we each create our own realities; communication is an essential part of this process whereby individual constructions of the world are created, and we often allow that construction which we have created through communication to control our behaviours in the context of future interactions. If, for example, we view ourselves as kind to others, and if this construct is a strong part of our self-image, we may attempt to act in conciliatory ways towards others at all times and in all situations.

The establishment of formal or technical definitions of communication illustrates well the difficulties inherent in this area. One listing revealed 95 definitions of communication, none of them widely accepted (Dance, 1970); a further attempt by the same writer (Dance & Larson, 1972) located 126 separate definitions of communication. In a general sense, Trenholm & Jensen (1988) saw communication as: '. . . a creative act initiated by man in which he seeks to discriminate and organize cues so as to orient himself to his environment and satisfy his changing needs.' More specifically, and with particular regard to the passage of information from one individual to another though the uniquely human communication modality of language, it has been said (Trenholm &

Jensen, 1988) that: 'Speech communication is a human process through which we make sense out of the world and share that sense with others'.

The numerous definitions identified by Dance & Larson each appear to be specifically directed to a particular form, or mode, or use of communication. As such, they do not go sufficiently far to provide us with a clear overview of the nature of communication as it applies to human behaviour within the broad context of the helping relationship. Trenholm & Jensen (1988) come closer to this goal in seeing communication as '. . . a dynamic process in which people collectively create and regulate social reality'. If a more concrete version of this is required, we can do no better than that of Schermerhorn *et al.* (1985) who wrote '. . . communication is an interpersonal process of sending and receiving symbols with meanings attached to them'.

Unlike many other phenomena studied in psychology, communication rarely has a definite or identifiable beginning or end, but is a dynamic process which is constantly moving and changing. In line with this process, whenever people communicate they form an interpersonal system. From this viewpoint, interpersonal communication takes place whenever two people become aware of each other. Then, each individual taking the mutual roles of sender or initiator, and receiver of information, they become themselves connected through the shared activity of creating meaning within an environment which may only be constant for the duration of the interpersonal contact.

All communication, of course, has an interpersonal element. Even in instances when two people are not interacting directly or personally, their interactions are partially interpersonal in nature. Communication by telephone, or more remotely, by mail, is still communication involving an interaction between individuals over time and in a manner facilitating the multidirectional transmission of information, such that the interaction, and its individual participants, are continually modified as an outcome. More simply put, individuals change as a result of communication, either directly responding to the nature or intent of the communicated message or, more subtly, as a result of the interpersonal interaction which allows personal growth.

The directionality of communication, as we shall discuss later in this chapter, is implicitly two way when communication is considered to occur within the interpersonal context. Communication involving the unidirectional transmission of information, however, must also be mentioned, if only briefly, to complete this overview. It might be said that the author of a book communicates by presenting information, in written form, and then making this available to others when the book is published and distributed. The communication here, of course, is not set within the context of interpersonal contact (unless readers of the book choose to approach the author in some way or other), and the direction of the communication is strictly from sender (author) to receiver (reader), with no mutual interchangeability of roles within the system. In an even more abstract sense, composers, painters, poets and others may be said to communicate, to the extent that they present a message, however it is formed or framed, and then make that message available to whoever might wish to receive it. In this sense, too, communication is definitely one way, with the receiver having little or no opportunity to reverse the directionality of the communication, at least not in any way which maintains the niceties of social politeness. For the most part, however, such specialized and abstract forms of communication (for the messages are not always readily apparent to the broad range of potential receivers) are the exception. The bulk of communication within the framework of human behaviour and activity is set in and is a function of inter-personal interactions of one form or another.

Within the nursing context almost all communications involve inter-personal interaction. Nurses are required, as part of their day to day function, to communicate both with their patients and their colleagues. In both instances, they are part of a complex social network, structured to a large extent by rules of interaction but open, none the less, to influence from each nurse's unique qualities as an individual. The nurses' environment presupposes communication through interpersonal inter-action, with even the simplest instruction necessary for nursing care passed from nurses to patients in a context of mutual interchange. And indeed, nurses who choose to disregard the two-way nature of that interchange, and to ignore the messages emanating from their patients, do so to the detriment of the patients.

Theories of Communication

Many different theories and models have been developed to explain the existence and function of communication. Lewis (1980) classified mod-ern communication models into several types depending on their context and function; these included the *technological, human behaviour* and *process models*. These are briefly described below.

Technological Models

Technological models of communication have been typically developed by engineers and not psychologists, and consequently individual differ-ences between sender and receiver are often ignored, assuming instead that these are fixed properties of the system, invariant in their function, concrete in their operation and fully open to objective understanding. Most often, technological theorists see the communication process as being straightforward and mechanistic. Although such an approach may be useful from an engineering standpoint, where communication systems are limited to circuits connecting pieces of electronic equipment, its usefulness in understanding the interpersonal communication that occurs between human individuals and within organizations is very limited. Technological models have little to offer to the understanding of communication within the context of nursing.

Human Behaviour Models

More recent theories, however (see Smither, 1988), have introduced the consideration of human elements that affect the communication process. These theories have placed particular emphasis on the characteristics of the sender and receiver as critical determinants both of how the message is sent (its content, form, tone, medium of transmission and so on), and how it is received (in a context of acceptance or rejection, by a receiver whose capacity to receive and make sense of information is clouded by pain or anxiety, and so on). Human behaviour models introduced the concept of a gatekeeper, or an individual who controls the information process. A gatekeeper determines what parts of a message may be passed on and what parts will be withheld. At first glance, the gatekeeper would seem to be the initiator or sender of a message, since it is he or she who first takes control of an act of communication. In face to face inter-actions, a sender will be influenced by environmental forces arising from the social context which shape the message sent to a receiver. The receiver will in turn, however, provide the sender with feedback, thus assuming a role of some influence in the overall act of communication. Nurses, for example, might be the initiators and, by implication, the controllers of most communications between them and their patients, but responses by patients, either verbal or non-verbal, and sometimes put in strong terms, will rapidly establish the two-way nature of the gate-keeper function. Human behaviour models of communication, therefore, introduced the cardinal importance of the human operators into the phenomenon whereby information is transmitted from one individual to another, and in doing so recognized the variability which these operators introduced into the system.

Process Models

It should be apparent, however, that the usefulness of the models discussed so far is limited because they view communication as an essentially static or inflexible phenomenon. In keeping with current thinking about organizations as adaptive and evolving systems with interdependent parts, most psychologists now recognize that communication itself is part of an ongoing interdependent system. Process models of communication view communication as a process involving interpersonal systems. Consequently, effective communication requires a constant adaptation to changing inputs.

There are a variety of process models of communication, but the following example, though the simplest, provides a useful overview of their various sequences and contents:

Source.............Message.............Receiver

This model indicates the three key elements in the communication process. Within the context of human communication, the *source* is responsible for initiating a communication by encoding an intended meaning into a *message* and then effecting transmission of that message through some medium or other (spoken or written language, other symbolic forms and so on). It is the task of the *receiver* to decode the message into a perceived meaning. Feedback from the receiver to the source may or not be present, but if it is, it may confirm reception of the message, allow assessment of the personal or emotional acceptability of the message, provide information on whether or not the message will be acted upon and, if desired, signal that the two-way process of communication should continue.

Consider the following example. The nurse, as the source, chooses to initiate a message that the time for the administration of medication by intramuscular injection has arrived. She therefore encodes a message to this effect, both by verbally telling the patient of her intention to administer the injection, and by appearing at the bedside with the necessary equipment. The patient may receive the message yet, by remaining immobile, give no indication that this has been so; communication may have been achieved but the lack of feedback provides no overt sign of this. More likely, however, there will be a visible signal that the message has been received, as the receiver (the patient) makes every sign of avoidance behaviour and then, realizing that this will not be effective in altering the situation, gives feedback in the form of compliance behaviour (rolling over to expose the required area) and, perhaps, a verbal component indicating the anticipation of pain and an appreciation of the inevitability of the coming procedure. The communication, for that is what has happened, may end there, with the patient choosing to suffer both pain and indignity in silence. Or the patient will frequently provide more feedback indicating a desire for a continuation of communication, usually in the form of behaviour soliciting words of caring from the nurse. Nurses may consider the process of intramuscular injection the most curious example of communication, but within the strict definition of a process model, that is exactly what it is.

Many recent communication theorists, however, have had some problems with models as simple as this since they consider, perhaps correctly, that the communication process is more complex. There are two major problems with many of the process models. First, as we have discussed in examples, it is problematical to treat communication as a one-way process and, second, it is untenable to treat the sender and the receiver as isolated individuals, devoid of the social context. The importance of the latter to communication in nursing is clearly evident when one considers the constant and complex social interactions which characterize the day to day activities of nurses.

More sophisticated models of the communication process have, therefore, been developed. It has been argued, in fact, that the communication process has five necessary components, these being (1) *source*, (2) *transmitter*, (3) *channel*, (4) *receiver* and (5) *destination*. Two early but influential theorists in the area of communication science, Shannon & Weaver (1949), introduced a further component, the concept of *noise*, defined as any disturbance that interferes with transmission of the message and obscures its reception by the receiver. Later this model was revised to include the concept of *feedback*, which attempted to deal with the fact that the receiver may not always receive the same message that the transmitter has sent. This model had a tremendous influence on the early analysis of communication.

A similar, though more recent model which serves to explain the components of the communication process has been reported by Stoner, Collins & Yetton (1985). Essentially, they argue that in the communication process a sender or source acts, as we have already said, as the initiator of the communication. Specifically, the sender encodes the information to be transmitted by translating it into a series of symbols (for example, spoken or written words) or gestures (for example, body movements). The sender is also, therefore, the *transmitter*, or at least the individual who commences transmission. The message is the physical form into which the sender encodes the information. The message is then transmitted through a *channel* represented by a number of different forms of transmission (for example, paper for letters or books, air for spoken or electronically transmitted words) in order that the message may be received by the receiver. Once the receiver has received the message, he or she decodes it, indicating that it has reached its *destination*. Decoding is the process by which the receiver interprets the message and translates it into a form that is personally meaningful. This model notes the importance of *feedback*, or the reversal of the communication process in which a reaction to the sender's communication is expressed. The factor of *noise* (that is, any factor that disturbs, confuses or otherwise interferes with communication and which can occur at any stage of the communication process) is also incorporated into the model (Figure 6.1).

Take as an example the situation in which the Director of Nursing in a major hospital wishes to inform her immediate subordinates of a change in the hospital regulations for administering analgesic medication, when required by patients, without direct instruction from the attending physician. She will be both the source and transmitter of that communication, by deciding on its content and then encoding it as a set

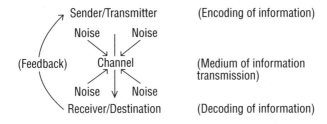

Sender/Transmitter	(Encoding of information)
Noise · Noise	
(Feedback) Channel	(Medium of information transmission)
Noise · Noise	
Receiver/Destination	(Decoding of information)

Figure 6.1 *Model of the communication process as reported by Stoner et al. (1985)*

of words. These words may then be committed to paper, as the channel, and transmitted or distributed to recipients or receivers (the charge nurses of each ward, perhaps), by whom they will be interpreted. Of course, since it is now the receiver's role to decode the message, this will be done in line with the decoder's own personal framework of interpretation, and may be done in such a way as to modify the original intent. An original message from the Director of Nursing which said 'Analgesic medication will not be administered except on instruction of the attending physician', may well be interpreted by the ward charge nurse to mean 'Analgesic medication should normally be prescribed by the attending physician, but when the patient is in extreme pain, it is permissible to give a little anyway'. This occurs simply because the charge nurse's approach to her work, which is that the relief of suffering is paramount, influences the way she decodes the message so as to allow the integration of this approach into her interpretation of whatever she receives. Coupled with this, the message from the Director of Nursing may come along with a dozen other instructional messages of various kinds, all to be decoded and interpreted at the one time, and the *noise* created by these other messages may serve to mask the real intent of the focal message. Thus, it is not surprising that in a busy environment, such as exists within a hospital setting, which is staffed by individuals of differing attitudes and approaches to nursing, the message decoded and interpreted by the receiver may not be precisely the same as that initiated, encoded and transmitted by the source.

The *source–message–channel–receiver model* developed by Berlo (1960) represents another example of a process model of communication. This model views communication as an interactive process, with no beginning, end or fixed order. The model does not allow for individual messages to be isolated; rather, they exist as part of a never-ending flow. Essentially the model lists five areas from which the source of communication arises. These in turn relate to the messages which are sent to the receiver. In addition, the means of receiving messages are the five senses. The receiver operates according to the same principals of communication as the source. Figure 6.2 presents a summary of this model.

General system theories, of which Berlo's is an example, also attempt to explain interpersonal systems of communication. Essentially, system theorists argue that whenever two or more people engage in interpersonal communication, they create a system. The relationship they create as the basis of this system is a unique whole, comprising in itself the complete means of communication between the participating individuals. As part of a system, each individual becomes interdependent, and changes to one individual, perhaps in the form of receipt and integration of information, will change the others either in subtle or more obvious ways. Nurses working within a team setting, for example, will form a communication system based on the interpersonal relationships which exist between them. When one receives information and passes this on to others, which is what communication is about, roles may change, activities may be set in place, expectations about the immediate and future behaviour of others in the team may arise, further information may be generated or sought out and further communications may be

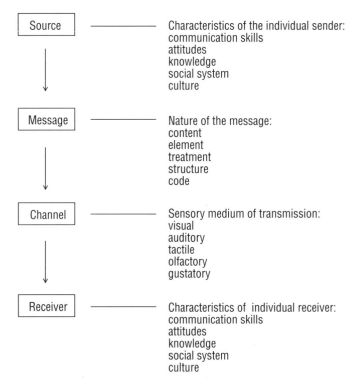

Figure 6.2   *The source–message–channel–receiver model of communication developed by Berlo (1960)*

initiated. Communication within a fixed, interpersonal system, therefore, becomes a dynamic process, having implications both for the function and the structure of the system.

An essential component of systems theory, whatever aspect of human psychology it may be applied to, is that the whole is greater than the sum of its parts. This means that when we want to understand a dyadic encounter (one between two people), we should not try to analyse what the members do when they are apart but rather how they operate when they are together. This interaction will be unique to the particular diad (or pair) in question. Its function cannot be explained simply in terms of the characteristics and communication capacities of the two individuals in isolation, but requires a complete understanding of the individuals, the uniqueness of their roles and relationships, the nature and purpose of the communications for which the system has been primarily set up and the potential involvement of other individuals and/or other systems in the process.

A communication system regulates itself in order to adapt to its environment by using feedback, or the process of comparing its present performance to a preset standard, and using this comparison to control its future output. Both positive and negative feedback are found in relationships where communication exists. If a relationship is going well, the partners will try to protect it from change through negative feedback (that is, feedback designed to discourage system deviation). At other times, positive feedback (that is, feedback designed to encourage system deviations) may be used to facilitate change.

In summary, recent work (see, for example, Deaux & Wrightsman, 1988) investigating and elaborating on the communication process has made the following conclusions:

1. Communication, in its simplest sense, represents an interaction between two participants, both of whom have speaking and listening parts to play. From this perspective, communication must be seen as a shared social system rather than a unidirectional channel.

2. As co-participants in this system, both parties bring to their interactions a set of expectations and understandings, or what have been called the 'rules of the communication game'. These shape the nature of the communications between participants. It is easy to demonstrate that such expectations influence communication. If, for example, you were asked to give an account of your views on the current status of nursing, its role in the modern world and the efficiency of its present organization, you may not respond in the same way to a fellow nurse (one of the same status and position as yourself) as you would do to the sister in charge of your ward or the Director of Nursing in your hospital. Indeed, the answer is likely to differ substantially given the different expectation you may have regarding the likely responses of your colleagues and of your superiors to the same message. For the communication to flow most

effectively, participants must share certain beliefs and suppositions that will enable them to coordinate their communicative efforts.

3. Verbal and non-verbal communications are part of the same system. Although it is sometimes useful to focus on one or the other, it is important to remember that communication takes place through many channels simultaneously. A person who is speaking, for example, is not simply emitting atonal words but words with a particular tonal message (soft, loud, angry, pleading, questioning, enquiring and so on); he or she will also be displaying facial expressions, standing in a particular way, and may be using a particular set of gestures. Sometimes the communications sent through these channels may parallel each other, conveying the same message, but at other times they may be contradictory, so that interpretation becomes more difficult. The nurse in charge of your ward may, for example, say to you in response to your question about when you can take a break, 'yes, you can go for your tea-break now', and since she smiles as she says this in a soft, relaxed voice, sitting herself at her desk casually looking at a magazine, you could easily interpret the message just as the words convey it, and go off for your break. On the other hand, she may say exactly the same words, but in a loud and hurried tone of voice suggesting annoyance and frustration, while at the same time holding a telephone in one hand to page the resident, frantically leafing through a patient's case notes with the other hand, and summoning the attention of another nurse with a repetitive nod of her head; under these circumstances, you could well interpret the verbal message as 'go and have your break if you must, but we are in crisis here and I am unlikely to be pleased with you if you leave us at this point in time'. The meaning is not, therefore, only to be found in the verbal content of the message, but in the tone and demeanour of the source (the non-verbal content of the message), and this is very much a function of the interpersonal relationship within which communication is embedded, and upon which it depends for its effectiveness.

As we have seen then, there are two major components of the communication process, these being the *verbal* and the *non-verbal*. We will now turn our attention to a more specific examination of these two channels of communication and look, along the way, at some further instances in the practice of nursing where these channels can be seen in operation.

Verbal Communication

Verbal communication is made up of discrete, separable units of speech, either spoken or written. It encourages us to create new realities and gives us the ability to think in new and complex ways. Verbal codes are also self-reflexive, that is, they allow the creation of representations of reality which may be passed on through communication, such that although the recipient of a communication may not actually have experienced a phenomenon or event, he or she may share another's (the sender's) experience by way of a description communicated through a verbal channel. Trenholm & Jensen (1988) have provided the following list of functions that language allows us to perform:

- to conquer the silent and the unknown;
- to express and control emotion;
- to reveal or camouflage our thoughts and motives;
- to make and avoid contact;
- to assert individual and social identity;
- to give or seek information;
- to control or be controlled by the world; and
- to monitor the process of communication.

Effective communication entails mastering language at three levels, these being semantics, syntactics and pragmatics.

Semantics

This refers to the study of interpersonal communication at the level of the word. There are two kinds of word meanings, namely denotative and connotative. Denotative meaning is public, conventional meaning. It is, in a sense, the meaning that was agreed upon when the language code was constructed, and is sometimes referred to as a dictionary meaning. Connotative meaning is a private, often emotionally charged, meaning. It becomes attached to words through experiences and associations. Here, individuals rather than the language system are the final authority. The word 'wart', for example, has a technical or dictionary meaning, that being a small, benign skin growth caused by a virus; for some it also carries with it the non-technical and private meaning of an unpleasant individual, unlikeable both in appearance and nature. Thus, to refer in conversation with a colleague to the 'wart in bed 4' may simply convey the technical nature of the medical problem suffered by the patient in bed 4, or it may convey, more privately, a personal opinion regarding the kind of person who occupies bed 4, irrespective of their medical condition.

Mastering the semantics of one's language is important, for no one can communicate competently without an appropriate vocabulary. Words bring about different reactions in all of us, and in order to utilize fully the vast power of language, we must be aware of the full meanings, both public and private, of all those words which we will personally use to achieve verbal communication.

Syntactics

This refers to the process by which words are combined and ordered into grammatical sequences. To convey meaning effectively in our verbal communications, it is important to be able to order or sequence words appropriately. Strict rules govern sentence construction and form. If we fail to abide by these rules we may well achieve negative reactions in others, the recipients of our communications. It is quite different, for example, to say to a patient 'may I roll you over in bed so that you are more comfortable' (syntactically correct) than to say 'may I roll over you in bed so that you are more comfortable' (syntactically incorrect, we hope).

Pragmatics

This refers to how we use sentences in actual conversation. Usually we use language to do things. The things we intend language to do for us are called speech acts, for example they can be directive, questioning, threatening, warning, requesting and so on. We know how to use language because we follow two kinds of rules, these being constitutive and regulative, which tell us how to understand and produce speech acts. *Constitutive rules* tell us how to recognize speech acts and *regulative rules* identify, in a given context, the speech acts that are appropriate and inappropriate. Speech acts are often conveyed in tone. The words 'time for this patient's medication' have quite different meanings when spoken in questioning and directive tones; the first seeks confirmation of an opinion while the second directs that some action should take place.

According to one model, the *co-ordinated management of meaning model* (Trenholm & Jensen, 1988), we have different rules for different contexts. In order for us to respond to any comment, it is necessary to consult a regulative rule; these rules determine the appropriateness of actions, given a particular set of goals and an understanding of the context within which communication is taking place. Pragmatic competence in communication is not easy, and embarrassment may result when contexts are misinterpreted or rule sets are inadequate. Within the context of nursing practice, pragmatic incompetence has the potential for quite disastrous misinterpretations of meaning and equally disastrous acts of omission or commission for the patient.

Overall, to communicate effectively, we must master all three parts of language, that is, semantics, syntactics and pragmatics. While all are clearly important, pragmatics bears the closest relationship to communication effectiveness.

Non-verbal Communication

The other major component of the communication process is its non-verbal form. Non-verbal communication is communication through facial expressions, body position, eye contact and other physical gestures rather than through written or oral expression. Although psychologists and lay people alike widely recognize that there is a non-verbal side to communication, we often underestimate its full importance. As we have already seen in examples of communication in nursing practice, the way a message is presented may convey as much meaning as the sequence of words which provides its formal structure.

Three conditions need to be attached to non-verbal behaviour before they are considered acts of communication. As Trenholm & Jensen (1988) have suggested, non-verbal behaviour must:

1. be perceived consciously by the sender and the receiver;
2. be intended as a definite part of the message by the sender; and
3. be interpreted by the receiver as an intended part of the message.

Non-verbal communication may perform several functions (see, for example, Trenholm & Jensen, 1988). First, non-verbal communication may convey how we feel about other people and how we see and interpret our relationship with them. It has been suggested that there are three fundamental dimensions of feeling expressed through non-verbal communication: liking for the recipient, status of the recipient and responsiveness towards the recipient (Mehrabian, 1972). We express these unique dimensions of a communication interaction through quite different patterns of behaviour. Our manner of approach, tone of voice, physical closeness, facial expressions, tendency to touch and general level of contact, for example, are quite different for someone we know personally than for someone we know to be of high status. A nurse's whole pattern of non-verbal communication would vary enormously between that directed towards a friend who happened to be occupying a hospital bed, and that reserved for the local bank manager who might come to occupy the very same hospital bed (at another time, of course). Second, non-verbal communication may modify verbal messages through a variety of means, such as complementing, accenting, repeating, substituting for and/or contradicting verbal messages. Third, non-verbal communication may regulate the flow of interactions, and especially the flow of verbal exchanges, by indicating to the other participant(s) in a process of communication, perhaps with a confused or frustrated look, or a hand gesture indicating a loss of meaning, that the output of information is too rapid for effective communication.

Patterson (1983) identified five specific functions of all non-verbal behaviours, these being:

1. to provide information beyond that carried by the verbal message, perhaps by indicating size with a hand gesture as well as with an expression of empirical measurement;
2. to regulate interaction — looking away, for example, to indicate a conflict of attention;
3. to express intimacy — touching a hand or placing an arm around a shoulder to add to or replace the verbal message;
4. to exercise social control — gazing disapprovingly at the sender of an unwanted or offensive message, signalling by this facial expression that its receipt has brought censure; and
5. to facilitate the accomplishment of a task — going directly to some purposive action following the delivery of a verbal message, to indicate that the whole message is directed at the achievement of action.

As a number of writers in the field (see, for example, Deaux & Wrightsman, 1988; Trenholm & Jensen, 1988) have told us, there are several major ways of structuring non-verbal communication. These are made up of the following categories:

1. *proxemics* (environmental preference, territoriality, personal space), all of which refers to the spatial disposition of the sender in relation to the receiver of a communication and vice versa, and covers the complete range of both voluntary and imposed characteristics of distance and position;
2. *physical appearance* (body types, clothing, artefacts), referring to the influence which directly observable characteristics of the sender and receiver of communications have on that process;
3. *gaze* (eye contact, expressiveness, regulation, looking or gazing in the direction of others) and *seeing* (visual contact with the whole person), bearing on the influence which mutual visualization has on communication between individuals;
4. *facial expression* (universal expression, facial blends, cultural display rules), having to do with the roles played, either general or culture specific, by the facial appearances of both the sender and receiver of a communication;
5. *vocalics* (vocal qualities, vocal characteristics), or the influence which tonal qualities of the voice has on the verbal message between two people engaged in the process of communication; and
6. *kinesics* (body movements and gestures) concerning the whole bearing of body movement on the process of communication.

Non-verbal communication is particularly powerful since non-verbal codes tend to cluster together to produce the same message in several different ways. For example, when a patient shows distress it will be indicated to the nurse (and, of course, to others) by the expressiveness of the gaze and the nature of the facial characteristics, the utterance of sounds with particular vocal qualities, and possibly by a form of touching and/or body movement, in addition to whatever verbal message is displayed at the time. These various ways of structuring non-verbal communication serve to modify the substantive content of messages, help structure relationships necessary for the transmission of those messages, and assist in the management and the flow of conversations.

Of all the forms of non-verbal communication, Deaux & Wrightsman (1988) tell us that eye contact or gaze is perhaps the most pervasive. People convey information by the amount and pattern of their gazing behaviour. A gaze can communicate liking, respect, attentiveness, competence and credibility, distrust, compliance or disregard. Gaze serves a crucial role in initiating communication and in maintaining a conversation once it has begun. For example, if a patient is looking around for someone to talk to about his/her problems and the nurse does not have time to listen, she will probably avoid eye contact. However, if she is able to spend some time discussing the patient's problems, she will most likely return the patient's gaze. Other messages simultaneously given, both verbal and non-verbal, may of course alter this simple equation; a message of distress or pain, for example, is likely to override the nurse's avoidance of eye contact and both enlarge and elaborate the process of communication.

Both Kleinke (1986) and Patterson (1983) tell us that gaze can also express intimacy in a relationship. People look more at people they like than at those they dislike. Gaze can serve as a means of controlling an interaction, or at least it often accompanies attempts to exert control. People gaze more at the receivers of their communications when they are attempting to be persuasive as well as when they are attempting to ingratiate themselves with the other person. Gaze can also facilitate communication between people who are working together on the same project. In an operating room, for example, some communications may be transacted and successfully completed primarily by an exchange of gazes. Clearly, the success of this will depend on the development of a closely shared set of expectations between individuals based on an intimate knowledge both of the people involved and of the context in which the communication is taking place.

In general terms, in the nurse–patient relationship eye contact or gaze provides substantial amounts of information. A person's gaze may transmit information that is not easily expressed in words. A patient's eyes may indicate fear or acceptance, or a variety of other responses to a nurse who is attempting to explain something or perform some function for the patient. Indeed, in those many situations when speech is impossible, a patient's gaze may be the major medium of communication. Simply knowing that these different channels of communication exist should make us aware of and better able to read non-verbal cues. It is important to be observant of the ways people use non-verbal cues and how they emphasize one particular cue in order to get their meaning across. Non-verbal communication is important in the practice of nursing both from the perspectives of nurse–patient communication and of nurse–nurse or nurse–other professional communication. Ignorance of non-verbal cues, or disregard of these even if they are perceived, will inevitably lead to errors of communication which may prove, quite literally, fatal for the patients under the nurses' care.

Barriers to Effective Communication

Communication almost always occurs through the verbal and non-verbal channels. Almost inevitably, there are barriers to effective communication in interpersonal encounters, that is, circumstances or situations in which communication is made difficult or impossible by disruptions arising in the sender, channel or receiver. A number of writers (e.g. Sayles & Strauss, 1966; Stoner *et al*. 1985) have identified common barriers to communication, and these may be listed as follows:

1. Receiving and processing only that information which we want or expect to receive — past experience leads us to expect to receive the same message in similar circumstances, and when those circumstances occur, we are only receptive to the expected information.

2. In a related way to this, ignoring information that conflicts with what we 'know' or expect to be the case — when we hear a message that disagrees with our preconceptions, we are likely to ignore the message, rather than change our ideas or seek some alternative explanation.

3. Making evaluations regarding the source of a communication — the meaning we apply to any message is influenced by our evaluation of the message's source, typically our evaluation of the sender and of his or her characteristics, relationship to us and the like.

4. Differences between the sender and the receiver in perceptions of the situation and mode of communication — words, actions and events are perceived in the light of the receiver's individual values and of the environmental pressures within which the message is sent.

5. Differences between the receiver and the sender in the meanings of words — words are only symbols of 'reality' and as such they may have different meanings for different people and in different situations.

6. Non-verbal messages which are inconsistent with the message content transmitted through the verbal channel — tone of voice, facial expressions and bodily postures can either help or hinder communication, but will invariably hinder it if they do not confirm the verbal message.

7. Emotional states of both the sender and the receiver — whatever

emotion dominates our mood (happiness, anger, fear, depression) will affect both the way we encode information for transmission and our interpretations of the relevant message sent to us.
8. Noise — the need to separate signal from noise and thus to receive a message effectively means that individuals will inadvertently 'screen-out' many of the messages they receive.

All of the factors listed above impact on our capacity to communicate effectively. Perhaps the most significant barrier to effective communication is noise. Noise is anything that interferes with the effectiveness of an attempted communication. Five special and particular sources of noise have been identified by research on communication. They are (1) physical distractions, (2) semantic problems, (3) cultural differences, (4) absence of feedback and (5) status effects. Examples of noise affecting the interactions between nurse and patient are common. Consider the following:

A patient is attempting to talk to you about the embarrassment he feels at having to urinate at the bedside. You continue to administer his medication while he tells you this, you talk to the nurse who is attending to another patient down the corridor, and you tap along to the music you can hear on a radio by another patient's bed. In this instance, you are suffering from physical distractions that create information overload. This constitutes noise, and as a result, your communication with your patient suffers.

A patient asks for a simple explanation of her condition. She is tired of doctors telling her what is wrong in a language which requires an encyclopedic memory. You, studying for your mid-term examinations and attempting to show how smart you are, provide the patient with a long-winded explanation about her condition, using a lot of big words you cannot clearly explain, thereby creating an even greater feeling of frustration in the patient. This is an example of noise arising from semantic problems which then gets in the way of effective communication.

You are treating a patient from a non-English-speaking background and find her difficult to deal with because she does not look at you when you speak to her or say very much in response to your questions. This is an example of cultural differences producing noise which then interferes with communication. The patient is not used to returning eye gaze with people she perceives to be in authority and so, contrary to being rude, is actually attempting to be socially appropriate in her interaction with you. An understanding of cultural differences may have assisted you in working through this difference and establishing more effective communication.

You are required to perform a task by the sister in charge of your ward, but you are not given the opportunity to discuss the task with anyone as you go about completing it. You know that you are on your own from start to finish, expected only to report the task's completion.

Upon completion, you are told that you have made errors and your performance has not been adequate. It turns out that there have been quite large discrepancies between your understanding of what was required and that of the sister. Lack of feedback has produced noise in the communication system and communication has broken down as a result.

You believe that a treatment schedule you have been ordered to carry out for a patient is incorrect or inappropriate, but since this has been ordered by someone in authority over you (the resident or sister in charge, perhaps) you are unwilling to raise this issue with your superiors for fear that it may be interpreted as criticism. The hierarchy of authority within the nursing profession has, therefore, created a further source of noise within the communication system, creating another barrier for you when attempting to communicate effectively. Status differences, whether real or imagined, can generate noise and so create barriers to effective communication between nurses and their patients, their colleagues and their superiors.

Despite these potential pitfalls, it is clearly important for each of us to be an effective communicator. In the helping professions such as nursing, this is an absolutely essential skill; without it, effective nursing will suffer in a multitude of ways. Failure to communicate effectively will lead to errors and mistakes, place excessive and undue burdens on crucial working relationships, increase workloads beyond their already heavy levels, give rise to personal frustration and anger, and ultimately may result in a diminished standard of care for the patients.

Being an effective communicator is both a natural and an acquired skill. Part of this skill lies in being aware of the process of communication and in recognizing and controlling communication barriers. Another part is simply to become good at encouraging the flow of information in your direction, that is, to become an 'active listener', and also to become good at giving constructive feedback in a non-threatening way to others. Fortunately, techniques have been identified and developed to improve communication and to overcome some of the barriers to communication we outlined earlier.

Overcoming Barriers to Effective Communication

There are several techniques which can be used by nurses (or indeed, anyone else) to overcome barriers to communication. Sayles & Strauss (1966) and others (e.g. Stoner *et al.*, 1985) have described a comprehensive range of such procedures which, if used correctly and effectively, may prove valuable in improving communication by removing barriers or limiting their disruptive qualities. These are the use of feedback, the use of face to face communication, development and display of sensitivity to the receiver's world, enhanced awareness of symbolic meanings inherent in communications, the use of direct and simple language in communications, and the use of an amount of redundancy appropriate to the situation and to the nature of the communication. Let us, then, look at these strategies in more detail to see how they may assist with the process of facilitating communication.

The Use of Feedback

This is crucial in all interpersonal situations where effective communication is the objective, whether we are using verbal or non-verbal cues to achieve this. Feedback is the process by which we tell someone else how we feel about something they have done or said, or about any situation in general which has involved a two-way interaction between us and another person. Giving feedback is particularly important when we are trying to communicate complex information to an individual not particularly attuned to the language or the concepts of the message.

If, for example, a nurse (the sender) is attempting to explain to her patient (the receiver) the cause of an illness, the nature of a medical procedure or the importance of a particular course of action, it is essential for the nurse to encourage the patient to ask questions and to indicate areas of confusion. By doing this, the nurse will not only be able to deliver a clearer message generally to the patient by clarifying issues, but may also learn to adjust her method of communicating to the particular demands of the situation, modifying and moulding her message to fit the patient's preferences and needs. In situations where a nurse is receiving information from a patient, she may use feedback to improve the process of communication by acknowledging, questioning and restating the patient's message as she interprets it.

At the same time, through careful and sensitive observations arising from more subtle forms of feedback, she may discover hidden meanings behind many of her patients' communications. For example, if a patient indicates an inability to handle a simple task which the nurse believes should not pose undue difficulty for the patient, this may reflect the fact that the patient believes the nurse has not been sufficiently sympathetic to the difficulties being experienced and would like more encouragement to perform the specified task.

There is, of course, an art to giving feedback within the context of the communication process (see, for example, Schermerhorn *et al.*, 1985). Specifically, it is important for the sender of a communication to give feedback in such a way that it is accepted and used constructively by the receiver. Feedback which is poorly given can be threatening and may become a basis for resentment and alienation. A nurse who says to her patient, for example, in the course of enquiring about symptoms, 'I think I understand what you are saying but please tell me again because I would like to be really sure', is more likely to end up with an accurate message (about the symptoms) than one who takes the first information given and declines to ask for clarification. The same nurse, responding in the same situation with that same feedback, is also more likely to maintain an effective communicating relationship with her patient than one who says to her patient 'look, don't waste my time with long-winded explanations; just tell me clearly once so that we can both get on with what we have to.'

The first requirement in giving feedback is to recognize when it is intended to benefit the receiver and when it is purely an attempt to satisfy a personal need. A doctor who berates a nurse in the operating theatre for not providing the correct instrument during a surgical procedure may actually be annoyed about personally failing to give clear instructions in the first place. Under these circumstances, though feedback is given, it is clearly inappropriate, gratuitous, probably offensive and unlikely to enhance the efficiency of future communications. Given that the sender's intent is always to give feedback which will be helpful to the receiver, it may be helpful for the nurse to remember the following guidelines when giving feedback to her patients (see, for example, Schermerhorn *et al.*, 1985):

1. give direct feedback, always include the patient's real feelings, and base the process of feedback on a foundation of trust between yourself and the patient;
2. be specific rather than general in your feedback, always using good, clear and preferably recent examples;
3. give feedback at a time when the patient appears to be able to accept it;
4. before giving feedback, check with others to support the validity of the statements you are likely to make;
5. give feedback only in areas that the patient might be expected to be able to do something about; and
6. do not give any more feedback than the patient can handle at any particular time.

Face to Face Communication

This is also an important way to break down communication barriers. Accurate feedback is nearly always achieved more efficiently through face to face than through written communication. Furthermore, people are accustomed to expressing themselves more fully and with fewer reservations when talking than when writing. As we noted from our earlier discussion of non-verbal communication, we are often able to communicate messages to each other through non-verbal as well as verbal channels, and face to face communication allows us to do this much more effectively than indirect patterns of communication. Therefore, use of face to face communication with patients is more likely to enable them to speak and act more freely. This is particularly important in many aspects of the nurse's activity, where patients are experiencing sensory difficulties or have significantly clouded consciousness, for example, and communication is often largely restricted to non-verbal levels.

Sensitivity to the Receiver's World

Clearly, individuals differ in their values, needs, attitudes and expectations, and this has a well recognized influence on the effectiveness of communication. Nurses, in undertaking their professional role, will encounter the full range of such differences and empathy with these differences will improve understanding of others and make communication easier. The stoic male patient, for example, intent on presenting an image of strong masculinity, will have expectations and attitudes regarding illness which are quite different from those of the elderly woman from a non-English culture, separated from her family for the first time, in pain and fearful of what is to happen to her. These differences in the 'receivers' worlds' demand quite different modes of interaction in order for communication to be successful. A blunt, perhaps jovial but patently factual manner, eminently suitable for the former, must be replaced by a softer, more overtly caring manner for the latter. Both patients are obviously in need of nursing care, but the differences in their backgrounds and personalities limit the modes of communication they are prepared to tolerate and respond to.

Awareness of Symbolic Meanings

Because different words acquire unique meanings for different people, sensitivity to these various meanings, even if they involve only subtle differences, can minimize communication problems. A patient may, for example, exhibit a phobia about the word 'operation'; some people, for a large number of unaccountable reasons, baulk at the word, showing all of the signs of anxiety and a strong desire for avoidance whenever it is mentioned. Simple awareness of this, a sensitivity to the distress felt by patients, and an openness to flexibility and compromise in minor details, is usually sufficient to counteract this situation. Under these circumstances, nurses are limited only by their vocabulary and by the dictionary they have access to. They could use the terms 'medical procedures' or 'curative processes' which the patient must undergo, rather than referring specifically to 'the operation'. Communication which might otherwise have failed because of patient avoidance can now proceed unhindered.

Use of Direct, Simple Language

Failure to do this is a frequent cause of communication breakdown and like awareness of symbolic meanings its correction is relatively simple. The more accurately the nurse's choice of words and phrases is tailored to the level of the receiver, the more effective her communication is likely to be. In dealing with a patient in a paediatric ward, for example, a nurse's language needs to be simple and pitched at a level a child can understand. The same adjustments must be made for adults from varying age groups and social or ethnic backgrounds. Nurses, and indeed most professionals, frequently forget that the language of their profession is a highly specific one, full of technical terms and jargon. This language may be largely unintelligible and quite unsuitable for effective communication with those outside the profession. Therefore, adjustment of language for communication with patients may require a special effort from the nurse but the result, in terms of delivering a clear message and ensuring that there are no barriers to effective communication, will be justified.

Using the Correct Amount of Redundancy

This is obviously important if a message is crucial or complicated, and if some form of compliance is required. In the day to day practice of nursing, it is often necessary to repeat messages in several different ways in order to ensure that the receiver will understand them. This applies both when the receiver is a patient and a professional colleague. Of course, caution and judgement must be used, and unnecessary redundancy or the overuse of clichés may simply dull the receiver's attention. Reminding a patient once that 'only two tablets should be taken once a day' may well improve communication, but repeated reminders can confuse the matter, particularly if the patient is on a complex medication regime involving several different substances. Similarly, reminding a colleague once that she has a particular duty for the day will, all other things being equal, probably result in that duty being completed; continued reminders, however, may only result in irritation, anger and an attitude of 'do it yourself then!'. A large amount of research evidence suggests that redundancy is less necessary in written than in oral communications.

Active Listening

A specific technique which can be used when attempting to prevent barriers to effective communication is known as *active listening*. This is a term which has, over the years, been popularized by psychologists and others in the health service professions, such as counsellors and therapists. It recognizes that when someone 'talks' or in some cases presents information for transmission in some other way, that person is trying to communicate 'something'. However, that 'something', the object of their communication, may or may not be what they are saying. The whole of the message, with all its subtle nuances and meanings, may not be fully evident in the verbal part of the communication. Part of the nurse's job in active listening, therefore, is to take action by helping the source of a message (the patient) to articulate what the message really means.

There are five guidelines (see, for example, Schermerhorn *et al.*, 1985) for active listening which, if applied by nurses in the practice of their day to day activities, will greatly assist communication between them and their patients. Nurses should:

1. listen for content of the message — try to hear exactly what is being said verbally in the message;
2. listen for the feelings expressed in the message — try to identify how the patient feels in terms of the message content. For example, is the message making the patient happy or distressed, and if the patient is distressed about the message, why this is the case;
3. respond to the feelings expressed in the message — let the patient know, sensitively and accurately, that his or her feelings, as well as the verbal content of the message, are recognized;
4. note all cues, whether verbal or non-verbal — be sensitive to the non-verbal as well as the verbal communications and seek to identify and clarify mixed messages; and
5. reflect back to the patient, in their own words, what they think they are hearing — restate both the verbal and non-verbal messages as feedback and encourage the patient to respond with further information.

The application of these guidelines, though seemingly simple, has been shown to improve communication measurably in a variety of situations, and their use in everyday nursing practice is likely to achieve the same effect. The importance of effective communication for nursing practice is self-evident; without it, patient care can only suffer. But awareness of barriers to effective communication, and the application of simple guidelines such as those we have reported and outlined here can remedy most situations where communication has apparently failed.

Summary

In this chapter we have attempted to explore the nature of communication, investigate its verbal and non-verbal components, assess the barriers to effective communication and explore the ways of overcoming these barriers. Communication is seen as an interpersonal process which requires an understanding of both verbal and non-verbal dimensions. While many potential barriers to effective communication are evident within the nurse–patient relationship, a number of ways of overcoming these barriers are readily available for the nurse's use. Feedback and active listening are two major strategies to ensure that barriers to effective communication can be overcome.

References/Reading List

Berlo, D.K. (1960). *The Process of Communication*. New York: Holt, Rinehart & Winston.

Bolton, R. (1987). *People Skills: How to Assert Yourself, Listen to Others, and Resolve Conflicts*. New South Wales: Simon & Schuster.

Bradley, J.C. & Edinberg, M.A. (1982). *Communication in the Nursing Context*. Norwalk, Connecticut: Appleton-Century-Crofts.

Ceccio, J.F. & Ceccio, C.M. (1982). *Effective Communication in Nursing: Theory and Practice*. New York: John Wiley & Sons.

Collins, M. (1983). *Communication in Health Care: The Human Connection in the Life Cycle*. St Louis: C.V. Mosby Company.

Dance, F.E.X. (1970). The concept of communication. *Journal of Communication*, 20, 201–210.

Dance, F.E.X. & Larson, C.E. (1972). *Speech Communication: Concepts and Behavior*. New York: Holt, Rinehart & Winston.

Deaux, K. & Wrightsman, L.S. (1988). *Social Psychology*. Pacific Grove, California: Brooks/Cole.

Duldt, B.W., Giffin, K. & Patton, B.R. (1984). *Interpersonal Communication in Nursing*. Philadelphia: F.A. Davis Company.

Epstein, C. (1974). *Effective Interaction in Contemporary Nursing*. Englewood Cliffs, New Jersey: Prentice-Hall.

Fraser, C. (1978). Communication in interaction. In H. Tajfel & C. Fraser (eds), *Introducing Social Psychology* (pp. 126–150). Middlesex: Penguin Books.

Fritz, P.A., Russel, C.G., Wilcox, E.M. & Shirk, F.I. (1984). *Interpersonal Communication in Nursing: An Interactionist Approach*. Norwalk, Connecticut: Appleton-Century-Crofts.

Goldhaber, G.M. (1983). *Organizational Communication*. Dubuque, Iowa: William C. Brown.

Hein, E.C. (1973). *Communication in Nursing Practice*. Boston: Little, Brown & Company.

Higgins, E.T. (1981). The 'communication game': implications for social cognition and persuasion. In E.T. Higgins, C.P. Herman & M.P. Zanna (eds), *Social cognition: The Ontario Symposium*, Vol. 1 (pp. 343–392). Hillsdale, New Jersey: Erlbaum.

Katz, D. & Kahn, L. (1978). *The Social Psychology of Organizations.* New York: John Wiley & Sons.

Kleinke, C.L. (1986). Gaze and eye contact: a research review. *Psychological Bulletin,* 100, 78–100.

Knapp, M.L. (1978). *Nonverbal Communicaton in Human Interaction.* New York: Holt, Rinehart & Winston.

Koehler, J.W., Anatol, K.W.E. & Applbaum, R.L. (1976). *Organizational Communication: Behavioural Perspectives.* New York: Holt, Rinehart & Winston.

Lewis, G.K. (1973). *Nurse–Patient Communication.* Dubuque, Iowa: William. C. Brown.

Lewis, P.V. (1980). *Organizational Communication: The Essence of Effective Management.* Columbus: Guld Publishing.

Mehrabian, A. (1972). *Nonverbal Communication.* Chicago: Aldine Atherton.

Mintzberg, H. (1973). *The Nature of Managerial Work.* New York: Harper & Row.

Patterson, M. (1983). *Nonverbal Behaviour: A Functional Perspective.* New York: Springer-Verlag.

Peters, T.J. & Waterman, R.H. (1983). *In Search of Excellence.* New York: Harper & Row.

Porritt, L. (1984). *Communication: Choices for Nurses.* Melbourne: Churchill Livingstone.

Porter, L.W. & Roberts, K.H. (1976). Communication in organizations. In M.D. Dunnette (ed.), *Handbook of Industrial and Organizational Psychology.* Chicago: Rand-McNally.

Sayles, L.R. & Strauss, G. (1966). *Human Behaviour in Organizations.* Englewood Cliffs, New Jersey: Prentice-Hall.

Schermerhorn, J.R., Hunt, J.G. & Osborn, R.N. (1985). *Managing Organizational Behaviour.* New York: John Wiley & Sons.

Shannon, C. & Weaver, W. (1949). *The Mathematical Theory of Communication.* Urbana: University of Illinois Press.

Smither, R.D. (1988). *The Psychology of Work and Human Performance.* New York: Harper & Row.

Stoner, J.A.F, Collins, R.R. & Yetton, P.W. (1985). *Management in Australia.* Sydney: Prentice-Hall.

Trenholm, S. & Jensen, A. (1988). *Interpersonal Communication.* Belmont, California: Wadsworth Publishing Company.

7
The Influence of Person Perception on the Helping Relationship

Living and working within any society brings with it a multitude of highly interwoven interactions between people. In all these interactions, we constantly form impressions of other people with whom we are involved. We do this in order to predict their future behaviour and to complete our social or other transactions with them as effectively as possible (Argyle, 1984). The process of forming impressions of others is often referred to as person perception (Hansen, 1984a). The ways in which nurses perceive both patients and themselves, the processes underlying the establishment of perceptions of others, and the consequences of such perceptions, once established, all have a fundamental influence on the nurse's approach to the practice of her profession. This chapter considers person perception in nursing, first from a theoretical perspective and then, through examples, demonstrates how person perception may be managed for the benefit of both patient and nurse.

Forming Impressions of Other People

We are often told that first impressions are important. Indeed, there is considerable evidence that people do make judgements of others on the basis of appearance alone. For example, when we meet someone for the first time, the most obvious information we have about the other person is based on their physical appearance. We are able to ascertain, more or less objectively, approximate height and weight, gender and possibly race. Somewhat more subjectively, we take in information on facial structure, expression and characteristics, style of hair, dress and grooming, the presence of deformities (a birthmark or an unusual swelling, for example), anatomical expectations that are not met (a missing finger or leg, perhaps), personal deportment and features of observable behaviour (cigarette smoking, agitation or calmness, implied threat and the like). On the basis of complex, detailed and divergent information such as this, all derived from non-verbal cues and without symbolic content, individuals derive perceptions of and make judgements about others.

A number of studies have been conducted to assess the impact of physical appearance on the ways we form impressions of others, and on the consequences of those impressions. Overall, it is difficult to over-estimate the effect of another person's physical appearance on our initial impressions of them. Not only are these physical characteristics a presumed source of information in themselves but they also serve as inferred cues to the characteristics of personality attributed to the individual possessing them (Deaux & Wrightsman, 1988). Moreover, impressions lead to actions which have a direct relationship to person perceptions. It has been shown by research studies, for example, that a person who appears to others as physically attractive is more likely than an individual perceived to be less attractive to be hired after a job interview, to have written work evaluated favourably by a supervisor or teacher, and to be seen by clients as an effective counsellor. Similarly, someone perceived to be physically attractive is also less likely than an unattractive peson to be judged by others, professional or lay, as psychologically maladjusted. By contrast, when an individual is perceived not to be physically attractive, that individual also tends to be judged to perform less favourably in most actions, and to be less competent and satisfying in interpersonal interactions with others (Deaux & Wrightsman, 1988).

We often form impressions of other peoples' personality traits from their physical characteristics. We might, for example, draw inferences of dishonesty, unkindness, gentleness or capacity for love simply on the basis of how an individual looks. In some very early and pioneering work in the area of person perception, Asch (in Deaux & Wrightsman, 1988) observed that in the process by which we form impressions of another person some items of information carry more weight than others. He referred to such influential characteristics as *central traits*. Prominent among these was the warm/cold dimension describing the emotional tone of a person. Asch showed in a series of studies that whether a person was judged by another to be warm or cold had a strong influence on further judgements which could be made of that same person. This central influence exerted by the warm/cold judgement was far stronger, for example, than the influence of other traits such as practical/impractical.

More recent research, however, has shown that the role of central traits is not as simple as Asch had originally argued. The centrality of a trait has been found to be dependent on both the quantity and quality of additional information that is presented about a person being judged (Wishner, in Deaux & Wrightsman, 1988). A person, for example, having been told by someone else that a certain person is warm or cold, may give less weight to this judgement if their own observations of that other person provide evidence of the opposite attribute; a judgement of warmth will carry less weight if direct observations show the other person to be unkind and rejecting, and similarly, a judgement of coldness will carry less weight if the person is observed to show kindness and acceptance.

In addition to the notion of centrality, the extent to which trait descriptions can be confirmed or disconfirmed has been found to be an important consideration. Rothbart & Park (1986) have found that traits vary not only in the ease with which we can confirm them but also in their ability to be disconfirmed. In general terms, favourable traits are hard to acquire but easy to lose, while by contrast, unfavourable traits are easy to acquire and hard to lose. To be convinced that someone was reliable, for example, may require us to observe that person for a considerable period of time, while to form an impression of an individual's unreliability may only take one episode of lateness for an appointment.

So far we have noted that observing a person's physical appearance and using these observations to make inferences about that person's character traits is an important part of the way in which we form impressions of others. In addition, however, the question of the *accuracy* of those impressions needs to be considered. As Deaux & Wrightsman (1988) point out, in order to decide whether a judgement about another individual is accurate, we must first have a reliable way of assessing the presence or absence, in the person being judged, of the trait under consideration. The literature describing the research in this area is, unfortunately, not clear. Of all the factors we might consider, the context in which we make judgements about others seems to be the most important predictor of accuracy. Clearly, people do not act the same way in every context; this is self-evident and frequently observed. It is possible, for example, to observe a colleague's behaviour in a staff meeting and form an accurate impression of him or her within that context, but still be unable to predict how the same person might behave at a party. In the same way, a patient, described as calm and compliant under circumstances of health, may behave in a totally opposite fashion when faced with the pain and fear of illness. The fallability of generalizing impressions of individuals from one context to another leads, as we will later discuss, to errors of judgement and to consequent difficulties with actions based on those judgements.

Citing the work of Swann, Deaux & Wrightsman (1988) point to the difference between *circumscribed accuracy* and *global accuracy* as the source of the problem. Circumscribed accuracy, according to Swann, refers to impressions that are based on specific traits that a person displays in specific situations. Nurses might, for example, be able to predict the behaviour of a loud colleague in a situation such as a workgroup discussion, where the specificity of the context provides a reasonably clear indication of the behaviours which might follow. Global accuracy, however, refers to an ability to form impressions of an individual that are valid across both situations and occasions. Extending the nursing example, global accuracy bears on the capacity to predict the behaviour of the same loud colleague beyond the verbal interchange of the staff room and in the home situation or, perhaps, at some social gathering. Extention of individual impressions beyond the context in which they were originally made, in other words, has pitfalls which must be considered if we are to understand fully the process and importance of person perception.

What is Perception?

In order to respond effectively to the behaviour of others it is necessary to perceive them correctly. As we have described in Chapter 1, perception is the process through which people select, receive, organize and interpret information coming from their environments. All skills, whether cognitive, motor or social, require accurate perception. To complete an abstract problem-solving task successfully, we require the accurate reception and interpretation of incoming information on which the task is based; this is perception in action. By the same token, to carry out a complex activity of motor coordination, like riding a bicycle, we must have full and continuing access to information on the world around us; without perception, we might rapidly end up colliding with the first part of that world we failed to perceive. The same is true for our interactions with other people; these are based on how we perceive the other, what impressions we have of them, and how they are judged in our eyes.

Through perception, we process information inputs of all kinds from many sources into decisions and actions. Perception provides a way of forming impressions about ourselves, about other people, and about day to day life experiences. But, as we have pointed out in Chapter 1, perception is not simply the process of information reception and sensation; it is also the process of interpretation, whereby incoming information is given meaning. Perception involves an interpretive screen or filter through which information passes before it is integrated into experience, and certainly before actions based on it are initiated and carried out. The quality or accuracy of a person's perceptions of the world around him or her, and of people or objects in it, therefore has a major impact on the nature and appropriateness of any decisions made or actions taken in a given situation (Schermerhorn, Hunt & Osborn, 1985).

Factors Influencing Perception

Clearly, since perception is such a complex process and involves a definite cognitive sequence, it can be influenced by many factors. Of these, however, the two most important categories of factors are those to do with the situation in which perception takes place, and those relating to the process of organizing perceptual information (Schermerhorn *et al.*, 1985). Of the situational variables which have been shown to influence perception, three categories stand out. These are discussed below.

The characteristics of the perceiver. An individual's background, values, attitudes, personality and so on may all impact on the perceptual process. Someone with a strong need for altruistic expression, for example, may seek out situations and perceptually emphasize aspects of the context that satisfy the desire for altruism. Negative characteristics inherent in the individual may also impact on perceptions. Negative views about group work may, for example, cause a worker to perceive unpleasantness whenever group meetings are held in the workplace. The nurse who may hold strongly humanitarian attitudes towards the relief of suffering, and have equally strong needs for independent action, could easily come to perceive the nursing environment as thwarting her own best efforts to help by channelling her activities into rigidly directed work patterns. This, in turn, may act to influence both her work performance and, ultimately, her attitude towards her profession.

The characteristics of the perceived. These too, may impact on the perceptual process in observable and far-reaching ways. As we mentioned earlier, for example, the physical appearance and overt behaviours of other people we observe in any situation in which we participate can influence the way we eventually perceive and define that situation. A doctor, espousing a position of authoritative knowledge about a patient, but dressed in torn blue jeans and having long hair, will certainly be perceived differently by other participants in the situation to a well groomed doctor espousing precisely the same position. The response which the nurse might have in these two situations could therefore easily differ. Though the level and accuracy of the medical opinion may not objectively differ, the perceived characteristics of the first doctor, as judged by the nurse, might easily result in less weight accorded to his opinions and instructions than those coming from the second doctor.

The characteristics of the situational context. These too have important implications for the perceptual process and for the ways in which situations are judged. The organizational and social structures in which we operate, for example, can influence perceptions both of situations and of the individuals who participate in those situations. The nurse who is asked to the supervisor's office to discuss ward policy or the progress of a patient will perceive and therefore judge this situation differently from one where the discussion takes place more informally in the tearoom, even though the substance of the discussion may be exactly the same. Situations involving structure and formality tend to be perceived as more important and therefore to be given greater weight than those occurring more spontaneously.

The cognitive organization of perceptual data also has an impact on the perceptual process. Specifically, there are a number of organizing tendencies which have been found to influence the meaning assigned to individuals and to the situations in which they participate. These are discussed below.

There is often a perceptual tendency to distinguish a central object from its surroundings. This is known in experimental psychology as the so-called 'figure and ground' response. As most of us will know from experience, there are some people who are noticed more than others in the workplace. Something about their appearance or presentation, their status and authority, physical characteristics, mannerisms, modes of expression or, indeed, their reputations, causes them to stand out from the background of all the other participants in the situation. They are, as a result, given special attention (whether positive or negative) and may be accorded special respect or prominence. But above all they are recognized as standing apart from the global situation.

Some individuals display perceptual 'sets' or tendencies to respond to situations in terms of anticipations rather than in terms of what actually exists. A nurse might, for example, having applied for the position of Area Coordinator of Health Education, be invited for an interview. The Chair of the interviewing panel, however, having read the applicant's file, or spoken informally with the applicant's colleagues, may arrive at the conclusion, prior to the interview, that the particular applicant is a poor communicator. Thus, despite an exemplary performance at the interview, with clear, articulate answers to questions and a logical exposition of health education policies and practices, the applicant might be denied the job, not because of her failure to display a capacity to communicate during the interview, but because the preconceived views of the interviewer incorrectly influenced her own perceptions of the applicant.

Some individuals display a tendency to assign an overall 'gestalt' meaning to events rather than experience the discomfort of having to deal with unorganized information. The term 'gestalt', as you will have noted in Chapter 1, refers to the almost universal behaviour of completing perceptions of situations based on predictions, even though the information available is incomplete. A nurse may note, for example, a number of her colleagues standing outside the hospital holding a discussion. Even though she does not have access to the substance of that discussion or to the context in which it is taking place, she may attempt to complete the perception by prediction. Thus she may decide that it is not an informal meeting of friends but a clandestine meeting of the staff union to which she was not invited and about which she was not informed. Her actions, based on this inaccurate but firmly held perception of the situation, could therefore be quite inappropriate.

People often demonstrate a tendency to try to understand the behaviours of others, or the events in which they participate, by attributing their causes to unknown but inferred environmental factors. The meeting mentioned above could, for example, be attributed not so much to the exclusive behaviour of a group of colleagues as to fears of a decision by hospital management to discontinue payment of overtime to staff. Once more, the attributed cause may have little or no basis in reality, and is most likely to arise from expectation, fear, incomplete information or heresay, but it can exert a powerful influence on subsequent behaviour. We will return to this point later in the chapter.

How We Understand Ourselves and Others

Perception is a crucial process for any nurse who wants to avoid errors when dealing with patients, colleagues or superiors, and this of course must be a dominant consideration throughout the practice of nursing. A nurse's response to a situation may be easily misinterpreted by a patient who perceives that situation differently. The same may be said of an interaction with a colleague or a superior. To be effective in their interactions with others, colleagues and patients alike, nurses need to recognize that perceptions may vary with circumstances, and they must try to take these into account when interacting with others. This involves having the ability to understand one's own perceptions of other people and situations, as well as the perceptions of the same people and situations which others might have.

It has been argued that in attempting to understand ourselves and other people, we all act as informal scientists, constructing our own intuitive theories of human behaviour and acting on these. As such, we face the same basic tasks as the formal scientist (Nisbett & Ross, in Atkinson, Atkinson, Smith & Hilgard, 1987), namely:

1. we collect data by making observations of others and of situations in which we and others jointly participate;
2. we attempt to recognize covariation in events and situations, attending to coincidences, co-occurrences and the like; and
3. we draw causal inferences about events and situations based on these data.

Observations

In carrying out these 'scientific' functions, we face the same difficulties as the formal scientist. When we collect data, we must attempt to do so in a systematic and unbiased way. However, this is not always possible. One of the factors that influences both the information we attend to and the information we recall is its vividness. Research has shown that our estimates and judgements both of people and situations are apparently more influenced by vivid information (information presented in the form of intense stimulation) than they are by information presented more blandly, even though the latter may be of equal or indeed greater reliability (Nisbett & Ross, in Atkinson *et al.*, 1987).

Moreover, even if we were able to collect information about people or situations in a systematic and unbiased way, our perceptions of those data can still be biased by our existing expectations and preconceptions (or theories) of what the data should look like. Whenever we perceive any person, object or event, we compare the incoming information with memories remaining of previous encounters with similar persons, objects and events. Such representations or memory structures have been called *schemata*, and are the result of perceiving and interpreting incoming information in terms of pre-existing mental representations of classes of persons, objects or events. The process whereby we search for the schema in the memory which is most consistent with the incoming data we have collected about an immediate experience is called schematic processing (Atkinson *et al.*, 1987). The concept of schema is, of course, very general, and has been defined as an organized configuration of knowledge derived from past experience which we then use to interpret our current experience (Deaux & Wrightsman, 1988), or more simply as a cognitive structure that helps us process and organize information regarding the present (Trenholm & Jensen, 1988, p. 57).

Research evidence on this suggests that the possession of schemata helps us to process information more efficiently and more effectively. Without the availability of schemata and the schematic processing which follows from it, we would simply be overwhelmed by the information that floods in on us from our constant interactions with the world around us. We would, in fact, be very poor information processors if we were not able to make use of this mechanism of experiential organization (Atkinson *et al.*, 1987).

In addition to schemata, we also have *prototypes* to help us categorize social knowledge. A prototype has been defined as an abstract set of features commonly associated with members of a category (of persons, objects or events), with each feature assigned a weight or importance according to the degree of association it has with the category in question (Cantor, 1981). More simply, a prototype may be seen as an organized set of existing knowledge that reflects the best example of a particular category (again, of persons, objects or events) (Trenholm & Jensen, 1988). Thus, for example, a particular set of characteristics will be linked to a particular category of people. We form prototypical images of movie stars (as wealthy, glamorous, exciting and aloof), barristers (as aggressive, learned, pompous and cunning), teachers (as intelligent, hardworking, underpaid and absent minded) and so forth. Nurses may, in fact, have their own peculiar set of schemata for particular categories of people, including doctors (as wise, authoritative, skilled and dominant), patients (as needy, complaining, troubled and dependent), or administrators (as narrow minded, miserly, rigid and constipated). We have, of course, taken these prototypic examples straight out of the air; they have not been established by any research study we know of. Having introduced the notion of prototypes, however, it is an act of personal instruction, and probably one of some enlightenment too, to examine what our own prototypes might be. Some insight into this personal realm of interpretation is invaluable in addressing, perhaps for the first time, what our individual preconceptions are when we encounter another person, perceive them, and make judgements about them.

As well as schemata of people, we also have schemata for events and for social interactions; such schemata are sometimes called *scripts* or *event schemata* (Abelson, 1976). A script may be defined as a coherent sequence of events expected by an individual, either as a participant in or an observer of a situation (Trenholm & Jensen, 1988). One of the most familiar scripts influencing encounters between individuals is the greeting script. When, for example, we greet an acquaintance with the phrase 'How are you?', our script typically calls for the response 'I am fine; how are you?'. This becomes an expectation which we carry into most if not all social or other interpersonal encounters. Having issued the greeting, we are therefore tuned to receive an expected response. When we are responded to, instead, with a long list of worries and concerns, we may be perplexed, offended, unsure of how to return the response, uncertain of the other individual and, therefore, cautious in any continuation of the interaction. Our expectations, in other words, have not been met, and we are called upon to display some unanticipated and additional information processing in order to complete the situation in any satisfactory manner. We may infer, rightly or wrongly, that the individual with whom we are interacting has failed to understand this very common social script (Atkinson *et al.*, 1987). But we may well be challenged by the need to reformulate a return of response which is no longer covered by a 'tried and tested' social expectation. There are many common examples of social scripts, each unique to the situation in which it occurs. Interacting with a sales assistant in a department store, for example, or with the electrician who comes to the house to fix a fault involves an expected script for social behaviour, and departures from that script necessitate information processing which we might not have anticipated.

What we must bear in mind, of course, is that scripts may vary not only by situation but by circumstance. The expectation that an open-ended greeting such as 'How are you?' will invariably be met with the response of 'I am fine; how are you?' may hold generally, but equally reasonably, the response may be replaced in some circumstances by 'Well actually, I have not been all that well lately'. An individual who has not been 'fine', has good reason to respond with complaint, particularly when the form of greeting specifically asks for a report on a condition or state of being. Nurses in particular will experience constant departures from the standard greeting script when they spend large parts of their lives greeting those who, by definition, have reason to complain when asked how they are.

Schemata, prototypes and scripts are actually mini-theories of everyday objects and events. All three concepts have been found to influence us in at least four broad ways (Markus & Zajonc, 1985):

1. *Schemata, prototypes and scripts may affect the initial coding of new information.* When a particular schema is activated by an object or event, it is likely to influence the way that object or event is interpreted by the observer.
2. *Schemata, prototypes and scripts influence memory.* In general terms, people are more likely to remember objects and events that are consistent with their existing cognitive structures than those at odds with or foreign to present memories.
3. *Schemata, prototypes and scripts influence our judgements, evaluations and predictions.* People generally anticipate that objects and events, when encountered, will fit their already established frameworks for understanding behaviour.
4. *Schemata may influence behaviour.* While this association is difficult to establish, it would appear that cognitive organization and interpretation of objects and events probably plays a major role in the determination of our behaviours in response to these objects or events.

In summary, then, our collection of data on objects or events is affected by our perception of the information arising from those situations. It is now well established by social psychological research that our strongly held beliefs about the world around us affect our perceptions of information in real life situations. Moreover, our theories of the world around us, typically based on past experience, shape our new perceptions of data arising from interactions with that world (Atkinson *et al.*, 1987).

Covariation

The second task we undertake when attempting to understand ourselves and other people is to explore what variables appear to correlate. Correlation, or covariation, refers to situations in which two things vary in relation to each other. The establishment of correlations is a fundamental task in every scientific endeavour, and has infinite use in everyday life. At a more or less objective level, we can state the existence of a multitude of correlations on the basis of available scientific data; for example, the number of times a patient has been to the hospital typically correlates with the patient's level of anxiety (though depending on circumstance, the direction of the correlation might be either positive or negative). As a general task, individuals attempt to draw such correlations all the time, usually without realizing that the process is taking place. Nurses have a particular set of correlations which many will recognize ('Southern European women report more pain during childbirth than Northern Europeans', for example, or 'female nurses are more caring towards their patients than male nurses').

Research has shown, however, that we are not very accurate in detecting covariation or in drawing correlations from our day to day experience. Our theories mislead us. In particular, it has been shown that when our schemata or theories lead us to expect that two objects or events or situations will covary, we tend to overestimate the correlation between them. We may even perceive 'illusory correlations' that do not actually exist except in our expectations. The nurse, for example, expecting that 'Southern European women report more pain during childbirth', may put into the case notes after a successful delivery that her Southern European patient was observed to experience considerable pain during that occurrence; the nurse may even recommend action based on that spurious correlation, by the provision, for example, of additional analgaesic medication. Conversely, when we do not have a theory regarding a perception of the world around us, we tend to underestimate covariations or correlations between objects, events or situations. We may even fail to detect and perceive a correlation that is strongly present in the data available to us (Atkinson *et al.*, 1987). Under such circumstances, the nurse, with no experience of hospital administrative meetings, and therefore with no expectations, may fail to detect the correlation between professional status and seating position at the boardroom table, thus committing what is perceived by the system to be the most grievous of social errors by sitting at the head of the table.

Causality

The third task which we undertake when we are attempting to understand ourselves and others is the attempt to discover causes and effects. In most scientific studies, the discovery of cause and effect is a paramount objective of the exercise. Similarly, in our personal efforts to understand human behaviour, we come to believe that we can only understand some instance of human behaviour when we know why it occurred or what caused it (Atkinson *et al.*, 1987). If a patient hugs her doctor, for example, the nurse may believe that her patient is truly fond of the doctor, or that she hugs all the medical staff. The former belief leads to an entirely different causal explanation of behaviour from the latter. In the first case, the patient hugs her doctor because she feels genuine affection for another individual; in the second, the hug may simply indicate a patient in need of affection or physical contact, or it may suggest an attempt to gain special consideration from someone she perceives as being a higher status member of the society. If the senior medical administrator of a hospital donates 10% of his annual salary to the establishment of a new hospital wing, does this mean he is altruistic, or has he been put under social or other pressure to make a gesture? We will let you draw your own causal inferences in this instance.

Attempts to recognize how we perceive the causes of behaviours (either our own or other people's) has become a major focus of research in social psychology. *Attribution theory* is the name given to the set of theoretical principles proposed to account for how people draw causal inferences about each other's behaviours (Trenholm & Jensen, 1988). The origins of attribution theory are to be found in the work of Heider (in Eiser, 1978) on phenomenal causality. Heider assumed that people are motivated to perceive their social environments, and the behaviours arising within them, as predictable and therefore controllable. He also assumed that the means by which we come to be able to predict events within our social environments is essentially similar to how we predict physical events; that is, we look for the necessary and sufficient conditions for such an event to occur.

Central to Heider's work is the distinction between *personal (dispositional)* and *impersonal (situational or environmental)* causation. The personal refers to the role we, as individuals, play in the causation of events within our social environments, while the impersonal concerns the influence of the situation or environment upon the causation of these same events. Clearly, this is not an 'all or nothing' phenomenon, and it is understood that some combination of personal and impersonal causes will always be responsible for the occurrence of events, though the relative importance of the two will vary from one kind of event to another. Since this early theoretical formulation, others have built on Heider's general distinction. For example, Kelley (1967) proposed three classes of explanations which we may offer when we try to interpret the behaviours of another person and has provided research evidence on the process underlying each kind of attribution. According to this evidence, as observers of behaviour in the context of social encounters, whether we are direct participants in these or not, we tend to account for another individual's behaviour in the following ways:

1. attribution of cause to the individual who is engaging in the behaviour (the direct initiator of the behaviour figures prominently in attributions of cause);
2. attribution of cause to the entity or individual who is the target of that person's behaviour (the recipient, too, bears some attributed responsibility for the nature and consequences of the behaviour); and
3. attribution of cause to the circumstances or the setting in which the

behaviour occurs (the environmental circumstances play a role, as well, in moulding the form of the behaviour).

Kelley (see also Atkinson *et al.*, 1987, p. 575; Deaux & Wrightsman, 1988, pp. 112–117; Trenholm & Jensen, 1988, pp. 70–71) argues further that in order to decide which combination of these three explanations of behaviour is reasonable we use three kinds of information, these being consensus, consistency and distinctiveness.

Consensus information consists of our knowledge about the behaviour of other participants in the same situations. In assessing this information we ask, in effect, the question: Do other participants behave the same way in similar situations? If, for example, all the nurses in a hospital left the building in response to a call from a union representative for a meeting in the car park, we would say that we had information reflecting a high consensus behaviour; if no one but you left the building, we would say that the information reflected a low consensus behaviour.

Consistency information consists of our knowledge about the participant's behaviour on other occasions. To assess this information, we ask the question: Does the individual behave the same way or similarly across a wide range of other situations? If a group of nurses leaves the building every time there is an industrial matter to discuss, this is high consistency information; if this has only happened once, we may conclude that it is low consistency information.

Distinctiveness information consists of our knowledge about the individual's behaviour among different entities or targets, or within different contexts. In order to assess this information, we might ask, for example, if a nurse tends to avoid only her superiors in the corridor, which we would term high distinctiveness, or does she take pains to avoid almost everyone, which we would term low distinctiveness.

Kelley argues that if we have information about each of these three factors, our causal explanations of objects and events will be quite predictable. Subsequent psychological research has confirmed Kelley's hypotheses. Particularly noteworthy is the evidence that there appears to be a tendency to overestimate dispositional causes; this is the so-called 'attribution error', and it is a point to which we will return a little later on in this chapter.

Errors in Perceptual Processes

While the methods we employ to form judgements of ourselves and others (namely, our attempts to collect information, ascertain covariation and infer causality) all provide useful tools to understand and predict the behaviours of ourselves and others, we need to be conscious of the many risks involved in the perceptual process. We make a number of systematic errors in arriving at our social judgements, and our inbuilt theories themselves often interfere with accurate information processing. Indeed, as we have glimpsed already, our theories can actually shape our perceptions of the data, distort our estimates of what goes with what, and bias our evaluations of cause and effect (Atkinson *et al.*, 1987). There are a number of perceptual distortions which might bear strongly on the appropriate and efficient practice of nursing, and we will examine some of these now.

Stereotypes

Earlier in this chapter we mentioned that as individuals we have cognitive schemata for different kinds of people. When you are told, for example, that you are about to meet an 'introvert', you will immediately retrieve your 'introvert schema' from memory in anticipation of the coming encounter. The 'introvert schema' reflects a set of interrelated personal traits which characterize an individual as reserved, cool, quiet and unresponsive. This schema will then be applied to shape the perception of the individual which you complete during the course of the encounter. *General person schemata* such as these are sometimes called *stereotypes*. Studies have shown that our schemata of classes of persons — stereotypes — are actually miniature theories of covariation. In the case of the 'introvert schema', the stereotype of an introvert is a theory of what particular personal traits or behaviours go with other personal traits of behaviours (Atkinson *et al.*, 1987). For this reason, stereotypes have also been called implicit personality theories (Schneider, 1973).

Throughout life and particularly through personal experience of interacting with the world around us, each one of us develops our own implicit personality theory, made up of a set of unstated assumptions about what personality traits (either in ourselves or others) are associated with one another. Such theories are considered implicit because they are rarely stated in formal terms and are often not part of conscious awareness. None the less, they dominate our perceptions and judgements of other people (Deaux & Wrightsman, 1988). As a general rule, people believe they 'know' which personality traits go together and which ones do not (Hansen, 1984a). As we have shown above, people assume that if an individual is described as an introvert, that person is likely also to be described as quiet, shy and unresponsive at social encounters. Because we are typically not consciously aware of the implicit association we are making between introversion and quietness, we are therefore unlikely to be able to notice any exceptions to this 'rule' of social perception and judgement.

Stereotypes serve an important function in assisting us to deal with the enormous complexity of the world we live in, and with encounters with people or events which arise from it. Because of our cognitive limitations (the extent to which we can process information in a given period of time) we are unable to attend to more than a small portion of the infinite number of stimuli made available to us by the environment at any given time. To attempt to cope with this, we mentally (though perhaps unconsciously) contrive to reduce the complexity of the environment. This may be achieved, at least in principle, by classifying other people and events into already known categories. The process whereby we then generalize back from categories of people or events to specific encounters with these people or events arising from our interactions with the environment, as we have discussed above, results in the formation of a stereotype.

Lippmann (in Deaux & Wrightsman, 1988) first introduced the term stereotype to the social psychology literature, describing stereotypes as 'pictures in our heads'. A stereotype occurs when an individual is first perceived to be a member of a group or category, after which all the attributes commonly associated with that group or category are re-assigned to the individual in question. A person is often classified into a group on the basis of just one piece of information (for example, 'introvert'), and then all characteristics commonly associated with that group ('introverts are quiet, shy, withdrawn and socially incompetent', for example) are reassigned to the individual. The difficulty with this, of course, is that what is true about the group as a whole (the stereotype) may or may not be true about the individual (Schermerhorn *et al.*, 1985). Typically, some characteristics may well apply to the individual in question, but to assume that the individual is the repository of all the stereotypic characteristics may be to ignore the uniqueness of the individual and misinterpret him or her.

In this respect, the related difficulty is that stereotypes often contain negative elements which, while applying to some individuals within a group, are unlikely to apply to all. Consider the example of racial stereotypes which abound in our society. A stereotype may hold that individuals from a certain ethnic background (it does not matter which) are typified not only by a partiality to food and song, but are also malingerers and use any guise of feigned illness to achieve medical attention and ultimately to gain compensation on false grounds. The former attributes are positive (who among us does not like to eat and sing); the latter attribute is negative. Nurses holding this stereotype will then be most likely to respond to patients from that ethnic background not just as fun loving people but also as people inclined to falsify reports of illness in order to achieve some gain. The whole pattern of professional behaviour of the nurse towards these people will become structured around doubt, disbelief and disdain and there will be a tendency to dismiss symptoms and complaints which might, in fact, be life threatening.

Two other common stereotypes which we find frequently in our society are sex and age stereotypes. The literature points to an apparently extensive tendency to use sex-role stereotypes on the basis of completely untested assumptions. The single piece of readily available information, that is, gender, often leads to such general and stereotypic preconceptions as 'women are always overly emotional', 'women are always unsure of themselves', or 'women can't make decisions for themselves'. The list of stereotypes based on simple knowledge of gender is seemingly limitless. Regretably, these stereotypes have consequences for behaviour within many professional contexts. Perceptions based on sex-role stereotypes lead to behaviours towards women, in particular, which may be totally inappropriate for the people concerned.

We may see, for example, a number of potentially negative effects arising from the operation of sex-role stereotypes within the nursing context. Women who express completely rational anxiety in the face of illness, for example, or well founded confusion over treatment methods because of the inadequate communication of information by the health professional, may unfortunately be simply dismissed as being 'overwrought' when they express this anxiety or confusion to their nurses or their doctors; women who are asked to sign release forms prior to complex and perhaps hazardous or painful medical procedures, and who express quite legitimate doubts about the appropriateness of the proposed treatment or about its value for them, may rather be seen as simply incapable of making rational decisions. The treatment which women receive in the professional medical context may easily vary with the sex-role stereotype held by the nurse or other health professional, and so women may not be treated with the respect that is their right within this context. The evidence suggests that sex-role stereotypes are not only held by men but also by women themselves, particularly if they hold roles of power and professional authority, and the gender of the nurse appears to afford no broad protection from the effects of sex-role stereotyping for patients.

Age is another basis for stereotyping within the nursing context which may have negative consequences for patients. Information on age, like gender, is readily available or easily inferred from observation. Many age stereotypes exist and wide (and sometimes wild) generalizations to any individual seen to be of retirement age or older can be applied. Like sex-role stereotypes, the possession of age stereotypes can easily alter behaviours towards older people in ways which challenge their integrity as functioning individuals. Categorizing older patients as 'weak, feeble minded, overly cautious and conservative, resistant to change, argumentative and dependent', as some of the common stereotypes hold them to be, may lead easily to distortions in how nurses treat these patients within the caregiving context. An older patient's request to bath himself, for example, though it will help him to feel independent and preserve his dignity, may be ignored by his nurses on the grounds that he is too weak, even in the face of contrary evidence that he is mobile and energetic. The concerns raised by an elderly patient about sharing a room with others may be seen not as a genuine desire for solitude, privacy and an environment which allows the pursuit of interests, but as resistance to change from old patterns of behaviour. These age-based stereotypes, and many others like them, while perhaps allowing greater convenience in the practice of nursing, can easily undermine the self-esteem of elderly patients who, through no fault of their own, require greater medical and nursing attention in their advancing years. Moreover, there is evidence that the loss of self-esteem and of the dignity that accompanies independence (or at least the semblance of it) may in fact contribute to the progression of illness and disability in old age, so counteracting any particular 'convenience' attaching to the use of stereotypes in clinical practice.

As can be seen, then, stereotypes obscure individual differences by allowing broad preconceptions to be generally but largely inaccurately ascribed to individuals. When this happens in the course of nursing practice, the nurse's perceptions of individual patients and their complaints may be rendered false and therefore unusable. Clinical activities subsequently based on these false or distorted perceptions may then go on to produce erroneous decisions in patient management, and can result in clinical errors of substantial proportions.

Positivity/Negativity Effects

The *positivity effect* is a general type of distortion in person perception which results from our tendency to form a positive rather than a negative impression of other people we see or encounter. We tend, in other words, to give the other person in our interactions the benefit of the doubt. Newcomb (in Hansen, 1984a) found that as a social phenomenon, people prefer to like rather than dislike others. There appear to be two factors which may account for this tendency. First, our need to feel secure in our environment could lead us to see only positive aspects of others. Second, we may assume a similarity between ourselves and others which is not fully justified in reality. Since most people have a favourable impression of their own personal traits and characteristics, there may be a generalized response tendency to transfer this favourable impression to traits observed in others. The positivity effect may therefore be based on an assumed similarity between ourselves and others (Sears, in Hansen, 1984a).

The reverse of this, the *negativity effect*, refers to the tendency of people to give more weight to incoming information on another person's negative traits than to information about their positive traits. You may recall that this point was raised earlier in this chapter, in the general discussion of how we form impressions of one another. Information about a person's negative traits has been found to have a greater 'modifying capacity' than information about positive traits. Modifying capacity (Feldman, in Hansen, 1984a) is the power of a trait, when paired with another, to change the evaluation in its own direction, whether positive or negative. Negative traits have been found to be more powerful descriptors of individuals than positive traits. It has also been shown (Hamilton, in Hansen, 1984a) that people are more confident of their impressions of others when these impressions are based on negative rather than on positive information.

Halo Effects

A *halo effect* refers to the situation when one attribute of a person or situation is used to develop an overall impression of the individual or situation. This is a process of generalization from one attribute to the total person or event. Halo effects are common in our everyday lives. When meeting a new person, for example, one observed characteristic, such as a frown, can lead to a negative first impression of a person who is, overall, considered to be 'cold' and 'difficult'. Like stereotypes, halo effects have the consequence of obscuring individual differences (Schermerhorn *et al.*, 1985).

Halo effects are clearly important in the nursing context since they can act to influence a nurse's perception of a patient's progress. Apart from using medical criteria, a patient's recovery or compliance with a medical routine is evaluated according to the impressions gained of the patient by the medical staff. As such, patients who appear 'well be-haved', 'compliant', and 'friendly' will be evaluated differently than patients who come across as 'difficult', 'resistant' and 'sour-faced'. The halo effect attaching to the former set of impressions (broadly positive) may well lead to an overall judgement of good compliance and progress, whereas the reverse may well be expected for patients judged im-pressionistically to possess the latter set of characteristics.

Expectancy (Self-fulfilling) Effects

The *expectancy effect* refers to the tendency to create or find in another situation or individual that which we expect to find in the first place. Expectancy is sometimes referred to as the 'pygmalion effect' or the 'self-fulfilling prophecy' (Schermerhorn *et al.*, 1985). Expectancy ef-fects relate closely to our discussion of stereotypes above. Our schemata influence not only our perceptions of individuals and situations but also our behaviours in response to these, and our social interactions in gen-eral. Our stereotypes can lead us to interact with those we stereotype in ways that cause these individials to fulfil our expectations. As a con-sequence, our stereotypes can become both self-perpetuating and self-fulfilling (Atkinson *et al.*, 1987).

Changes in our own behaviour, resulting from an impression of another person, can, in social interaction, alter the other person's behaviour so that it confirms the impression (Hansen, 1984a). If, for example, we have formed an impression of someone else as an insensitive person, we are then prone to emphasize in perceptions of the other person those behaviours we see as consistent with insensitivity. We may also change our own behaviours in accord with this overall situation. We might, for example, adopt an impolite or rude approach to that person, simply because this approach confirms our perceptions of their own characteristics. The other person, then being aware of our rudeness, may become gruff in reply. Because we assume that gruffness and insensitivity go together, we come to believe that our interpretation is thus the correct one. Our impression of another individual, through our own behaviour towards that individual, has therefore become self-fulfilling.

Self-fulfilling effects can have both positive and negative outcomes for nurses. A nurse may believe, for example, that all patients diagnosed as HIV positive are only marginally committed to the treatment program they are currently undertaking, and therefore do not require any specialist counselling (as other patient groups suffering from potentially terminal states, for example cancer patients, typically receive at the hospital). The consequences of this for the HIV-positive patient group might well be, therefore, a real decline in commitment to the treatment program. This will then confirm the nurse's earlier view in a circular process which could have dire consequences for her patients. For some patients, involvement in any form of treatment, though perhaps necessary, is something they would like to avoid thinking about, and they might therefore welcome the lack of interest or involvement shown by the nursing staff. For other patients, however, this may be a disappointing outcome since they may have welcomed the establishment of a therapeutic or support group attending to their psychological and social needs to complement the medical treatment.

Fundamental Attribution Error

Earlier in this chapter, we mentioned the phenomenon known as the *attribution problem* (the task of attempting to infer the causes of behaviour). Since attribution is the process of inferring causality, it is also one of the main means by which people organize perceptual data about other individuals, objects or situations (Schermerhorn *et al.*, 1985). One of the major attribution tasks we face daily in the process of person perception is that of deciding whether an observed behaviour reflects something unique about the person (his or her attitudes, personality characteristics and the like), or something about the situation in which we observe the person (cold, friendly, forced and the like). If we infer that something about the person (some observable or assumed characteristic) is primarily responsible for their behaviour, then our inference is called an internal or dispositional attribution (disposition refers to a person's beliefs, attitudes and personality characteristics). If, however, we conclude that some external cause is primarily responsible for their behaviour (for instance, threat of punishment, or promise of financial gain, perhaps), it is called an external or situational attribution (Atkinson *et al.*, 1987).

Heider (in Atkinson *et al.*, 1987, p. 577), the founder of modern attribution theory, noted that an individual's behaviour is so compelling to observers that they take it at face value, so giving insufficient weight to the circumstances surrounding it. As we have mentioned above, recent research has confirmed Heider's speculation. We, as individuals, typically underestimate the situational causes of behaviour in others, jumping too easily to conclusions about the dispositions (internal characteristics) of that other person. Argyle (1984) found that one of the most widespread errors in forming impressions of other people, and one which should be particularly avoided by those who work in a service delivery role with other people, is assuming that another individual's behaviour is mainly a product of 'personality', that is, of internal, preordained and unchangeable traits or characteristics. In fact, much of human behaviour, as contemporary psychological research continues to reveal, is more a function of situation than of enduring 'personality' traits. Atkinson *et al.* (1987, p. 577) put it this way: 'We (in Western society, at any rate) have a schema of cause and effect in human behaviour that gives too much weight to the person and too little to the situation'. This bias toward dispositional rather than situational attributions has been termed the *fundamental attribution error* (Ross, in Atkinson *et al.*, 1987, p. 577).

It is important to recognize that the mistakes we make when forming impressions of other people are the same sorts of mistakes we make in our own self-perceptions. Understanding ourselves is one of our major tasks as informal scientists going about the job of living within a society, and it would seem that we make judgements about ourselves by using the same inferential processes and making the same inferential errors that we use for making judgements about others (Bem, 1972). When we attempt to understand our own behaviour, we also commit the fundamental attribution error. We make dispositional attributions when we should, in the interests of perceptual accuracy, be making situational attributions.

The tendency to accept greater personal responsibility for positive outcomes than for negative outcomes has also been noted in the literature and has been termed the *self-serving attribution bias*. Zuckerman (1979) deduced from a survey of the available research literature that there was a tendency for people to claim that success on a task was due to personal ability or to the amount of effort they exerted. These are, of course, qualities associated with individuals themselves. People are much more likely to seek situational causes why they fail in some task, preferring to look outside themselves for an explanation. The self-serving bias is also in evidence when people estimate the magnitude of their own influence on outcomes of other peoples' 'tasks'. While nurses may, for example, claim that their own efforts were largely responsible for their patients' recoveries, they are less likely to take personal responsibilities for their failures, preferring instead to look towards situational explanations to account for the more negative aspects of outcomes.

Summary

It can be seen that in forming judgements of ourselves and other people, we make a number of widespread errors. It is important for those of us working with people in the health care professions to recognize the ubiquitous nature of distortions in the perceptions we make both of other people and of situations, and to make every effort to avoid forming impressions of others which are based on such widespread, well recognized and easily avoided biases.

In this chapter we have attempted to explain the process of person perception. We began by considering the manner in which we form impressions of others. It was argued that we tend to use a scientific model in our efforts to construct our theories of human behaviour based on our observations of others. The ways in which we collect data, detect covariation and infer causality were considered. The principal types of perceptual distortions which confront all of us when we are forming impressions of ourselves and others were also considered, and examples of relevance to nursing practice were given.

References/Reading List

Abelson, R.P. (1976). Script processing in attitude formation and decision making. In J.S. Carroll & J.W. Payne (eds), *Cognition and Social Behavior*. Hillsdale, New Jersey: Erlbaum.

Argyle, M. (1984). Social behaviour. In C.L. Cooper & P. Makin, (eds), *Psychology for Managers*. Trowbridge, Wiltshire: Macmillan.

Atkinson, R.L., Atkinson, R.C., Smith, E.E. & Hilgard, E.R. (1987). *Introduction to Psychology*. San Diego: Harcourt Brace Jovanovich.

Bem, D.J. (1972). Self perception theory. In L. Berkowitz (ed.), *Advances in Experimental Social Psychology*, Vol. 6. New York: Academic Press.

Cantor, N. (1981). A cognitive-social approach to personality. In N. Cantor & J.F. Kihlstrom (eds), *Personality, Cognition and Social Interaction*. Hillsdale, New Jersey: Erlbaum.

Deaux, K. & Wrightsman, L.S. (1988). *Social Psychology*. Pacific Grove, California: Brooks/Cole.

Eiser, J.R. (1978). Interpersonal attributions. In H. Tajfel & C. Fraser (eds), *Introducing Social Psychology*. Middlesex: Penguin.

Hansen, R.D. (1984a). Person perception. In A.S. Kahn (ed.), *Social Psychology*. Dubuque, Iowa: William C. Brown.

Hansen, R.D. (1984b). Attribution. In A.S. Kahn (ed.), *Social Psychology*. Dubuque, Iowa: William C. Brown.

Hilgard, E.R., Atkinson, R.C. & Atkinson, R.L. (1975). *Introduction to Psychology*. New York: Harcourt Brace Jovanovich.

Hollander, E.P. (1976). *Principles and Methods of Social Psychology*. New York: Oxford University Press.

Katz, D. & Kahn, R.L. (1978). *The Social Psychology of Organizations*. New York: John Wiley & Sons.

Kelley, H.H. (1967). Attribution theory in social psychology. In D. Levine (ed.), *Nebraska Symposium on Motivation*, 15, 192–238.

Lindzey, G. & Aronson, E. (eds) (1985). *Handbook of Social Psychology*. New York: Random House.

Markus, H. & Zajonc, R.B. (1985). The cognitive perspective in social psychology. In G. Lindzey & E. Aronson (eds), *Handbook of Social Psychology*. New York: Random House.

Newcomb, T.M., Turner, R.H. & Converse, P.E. (1969). *Social Psychology: The Study of Human Interaction*. London: Routledge & Kegan Paul.

Ross, L. (1977). The intuitive psychologist and his shortcomings: distortions in the attribution process. In L. Berkowitz (ed.), *Advances in Experimental Social Psychology*, Vol. 10. New York: Academic Press.

Rothbart, M. & Park, B. (1986). On the confirmability and disconfirmability of trait concepts. *Journal of Personality and Social Psychology*, 50, 131–142.

Schermerhorn, J.R., Hunt, J.G. & Osborn, R.N. (1985). *Managing Organizational Behavior*. New York: John Wiley & Sons.

Schneider, D.J. (1973). Implicit personality theory: a review. *Psychological Bulletin*, 79, 294–309.

Swann, W.B. (1984). Quest for accuracy in person perception: a matter of pragmatics. *Psychological Review*, 91, 457–477.

Trenholm, S. & Jensen, A. (1988). *Interpersonal Communication*. Belmont, California: Wadsworth Publishing Company.

Zuckerman, M. (1979). Attribution of success and failure revisited, or: the motivational bias is alive and well in attribution theory. *Journal of Personality*, 47, 245–287.

8
Group Processes and the Practice of Nursing

A vast array of human behaviours, including many if not all of the helping behaviours, are to be seen only within groups. Consequently, psychologists have become interested in such things as the structure of human groups, how these groups form, the process of group decision making, and patterns of group leadership. Groups are so pervasive within our society that sometimes it is difficult to identify exactly what to study. Groups may form because of friendship, profession, physical proximity, race, gender, religion, or indeed virtually any other category of individual characteristic or situation we can think of. They can consist of just a few people or thousands (Smither, 1988).

In this chapter we will consider and define the notion of groups and examine their types, formation and characteristics. In addition, we will look at the nature of group decision-making processes and set out the applications of certain therapeutic groups within the practice of nursing. Given the importance of group structure and behaviour to nursing practice, we will also consider the personal characteristics and skills necessary for the effective leadership of specific groups that nurses might use as part of their daily activities.

Defining Groups

It is virtually impossible to avoid being a member of some group or other. Typically, we belong to many groups, some interrelated, others independent. A person may, for example, be an Australian citizen, come from a Chinese background, play in a softball team, work in the profession of nursing and belong to an extended network of family and friends. At any given moment, some of these groups will have more influence on the person than others, and at that time the individual is likely to adapt his or her behaviour to fit the standards and expectations of the group with which he or she is at present identifying (Deaux & Wrightsman, 1988; Smither, 1988).

The first task which psychologists face when studying group behaviour is to identify the structural boundaries of the group to be studied (Smither, 1988). McGrath (in Deaux & Wrightsman, 1988) gives the following working definition of groups: 'A group is an aggregation of two or more people who are to some degree in dynamic interrelation with one another'. More formally, Wexley & Yukl (in Schermerhorn, Hunt & Osborn, 1985, pp. 245–46) have defined a group as: 'a collection of people who interact with each other regularly over a period of time and see themselves to be mutually dependent with respect to the attainment of one or more common goals'. The key elements which we may distil from these definitions are *interaction, time* and *feelings of mutual dependence for goal accomplishment.* Groups differ from simple aggregates of individuals in several respects. In contrast to groups, the term aggregate refers merely to collections of individuals who do not interact with one another in the ways outlined above. People waiting for a bus typically do not interact with one another except in the totally superficial way that sheer physical proximity imposes; nor do they share feelings to such a degree that they may influence one another's behaviours or thoughts. Such collections of people would not, therefore, meet the criteria necessary for the establishment of groups (Deaux & Wrightsman, 1988).

Whereas an aggregate has no particular structure, a group has some definite form of organization, and its members have some relationship with one another, albeit broadly based. Groups are dynamic or interactive in their existence and function, whereas aggregates are largely passive. Members of groups are aware of one another, of each other's behaviours and of the purpose of the group, while people in an aggregate are usually oblivious of others, who simply happen to share the same space at the same time (Deaux & Wrightsman, 1988).

Schein (in Schermerhorn *et al.*, 1985) has referred to the concept of *psychological groups*, meaning that in addition to the criteria set out above for group structure, group members are also aware of what each other member needs from the group, and the contributions each might make to it. Of course, not all groups are psychological groups, and the focus in this chapter will be on groups *per se* rather than psychological ones.

Types of Groups

Primary/Informal Groups

Primary or informal groups typically arise outside conventional organizational structures. These groups may use a common task as a basis for their formation; several nurses engaged in the shared activity of changing a patient's dressing, for example, would, for the duration of that task, constitute a primary or informal group. But many other factors can lead to the formation of these groups. Primary or informal groups may also, for example, be organized along the lines of social class, ethnic background or friendship. A collection of nurses choosing, because of personal liking and shared values, to meet outside the occupational setting to go bowling, see a movie or simply meet and talk over coffee, would constitute a clear-cut primary or informal group. Primary or informal groups are, therefore, characterized by an absence of formality in their structure and formation, by shared values among members, and by a concern for mutual friendship or welfare. Primary or informal groups exist without being formally established or specified by someone in authority, and are often found as subgroups within more formal groups. It will be clear from this that primary or informal groups develop between, as well as within, groups at all levels within the workplace (Smither, 1988; Schermerhorn *et al.*, 1985). There is considerable scope for the formation of such groups within the context of nursing practice, and even the most cursory scrutiny of your own occupational settings and activities will reveal many examples of such groups, often transient but always functional in their intent and formation.

Secondary/Formal Groups

Secondary or formal groups tend to be created through the operation (and perhaps the imposition) of some formal authority, and their establishment comes about for some particular premeditated or preordained purpose. They typically centre on quite clear-cut interpersonal relationships, usually involving individuals in formally designated roles of superiority or authority (perhaps by reason of their skills, training or experience) and others in equally designated roles of a more subordinate kind (often arising from their more junior status), where the former provide direction and the latter follow instructions. Moreover, they are firmly characterized by having group tasks and leaders chosen by some higher management structure or individual.

These groups tend to have formal rules of operation directed towards the achievement of some prior specified outcome, behaviour within them is generally impersonal and unspontaneous and follows an established and largely invariant pattern, and they often appear on formal organizational charts of occupational groups (Smither, 1988; Schermerhorn *et al.*, 1985). Within the nursing context, a single shift comprising a set number of nurses arranged in a hierarchy of authority, with each individual having set tasks and established and expected ways of accomplishing these tasks, with the whole 'group' lasting only for a predetermined period of time (the duration of the shift), would provide an example of a secondary or formal group.

The key difference between primary/informal and secondary/formal groups is that the former emerge spontaneously, whereas the latter are designated by some overriding organizational authority. While a specific occupational task is usually the basis for the formation of a secondary group, friendship or the sharing of personal characteristics is likely to be more important in the formation of a primary group. Although primary or informal groups do not appear on organizational charts setting out occupational or other groups, they can have a powerful influence on such areas as organizational dynamics, employee morale and worker productivity (Smither 1988; Schermerhorn *et al.*, 1985). A primary or informal group of nurses, for example, joined by friendship or shared characteristics of one kind or another, can work to cement the functioning of a secondary or formal group and improve its efficiency, if its members agree with its objectives and respect the hierarchy which put it into place. If they do not, however, the same primary or informal group can work quite effectively towards the collapse of the more formal structure. Many instances, from informal group activity directed towards winning the monthly hospital ward efficiency award to activities of the same group involved in a major industrial dispute, show the power of informal groups within more formal group structures, and nursing and other medical administrators ignore this well established phenomenon at their peril.

There are at least two reasons why informal groups emerge to co-exist with formal groups in organizations or in occupational settings. First, they help people perform their jobs more effectively and efficiently. Informal groups offer a network of interpersonal relationships with the potential to assist the work flow in ways that formal lines of authority may fail to provide. Formal groups of nurses (a single shift on a ward, for example) may have a broad, well established and rule-bound function to perform, but the formation of informal groups in response to specific demands (two nurses mutually assisting one another with a procedure for an individual patient, for example) adds immeasurable efficiency and effectiveness to the overall, organization-determined work plan. Second, informal groups help individuals to satisfy personal needs that may be largely unmet in a person's formal group affiliations. Informal groups provide opportunities (1) to develop friendships and companionships from within the broader organizational or occupational setting, (2) to find sympathy for one's feelings and confirmation with one's actions in the face of professional alienation and uncertainty, (3) to find help and assistance with specific difficulties from people other than one's formal superior (with whom there may be communication difficulties based on perceptions of status), and (4) to achieve a sense of belonging with people who share similar values, attitudes and goals (Schermerhorn *et al.*, 1985).

Group Formation

Formal Groups

Since newly formed groups show quite different behaviour patterns from mature ones, it is important to know the stage of development of a given group in order to understand that group and assess its effectiveness. This knowledge enables us to predict the kinds of behaviour most likely to occur within groups at different stages of development, and to understand why groups act in quite different ways. A synthesis of the extensive psychological research on small groups suggests that there are four distinct phases of group development, these being (1) *forming*, (2) *storming*, (3) *initial integration* (or *norming*), and (4) *total integration* (or *performing*) (Tuckman, 1965; see Smither, 1988, and Schermerhorn *et al.*, 1985). The available research suggests that these particular stages of group development are characteristic of secondary/ formal groups rather than of primary/informal groups.

The forming stage of formal groups involves the initial entry of individual members into the group. In the forming stage, people wish to ascertain what is acceptable behaviour and what the real task of the group is. During the forming stage, the issue of the relative status of group members is unclear and needs to be confronted. For example, although most work groups might have a designated head, real power may in fact lie in other members. During the first stage of group formation, social interaction tends to be limited as members focus mostly on the task to be accomplished.

The second stage of group development is a period of high emotionality. Typically, the storming period involves relatively high tension among the members involving periods of overt hostility and infighting. Noticeable changes occur in the group at this stage. Specifically, as the group moves into the storming stage, some negative behaviour is seen to occur among many members of the group as they begin to establish positions of status within the group. This often involves both hostile and acrimonious verbal exchanges. Certain individuals begin to establish themselves as leaders of the group, and at the same time, other assertive members may challenge this newly established leadership. The storming stage lasts until the status hierarchy within the group is relatively well established.

While the storming phase is characterized by differences among group members, the norming phase of group development is concerned with integration of structures and roles within the group. Once the status of each member is determined (during storming), the group enters the initial integration or norming stage and it is at this point that the group sets standards for behaviour and develops ways for working together. Members are likely to develop a sense of closeness (real or imagined), a workable communication network, a clear division of labour and norms for group behaviour designed to protect the group from disintegration.

Finally, the group moves toward the total integration or performing stage. Total integration characterizes a mature, organized and well functioning group. The integration is now completed. The group is able to address problems to be solved or tasks to be accomplished. In addition, the group is able to handle membership disagreements or disputes about group behaviour and functioning in creative and adaptive ways. As the group moves from the forming stage to the total integration (or performing) stage, the amount of purely informational, functional or task oriented communication declines, and communication for social purposes increases. After a group decision has been reached, and behaviours are initiated which are directed towards putting that decision into place, members engage in considerably more social interaction than they had previously felt free to undertake.

To place this process into context, consider the processes of group formation which might take place if a hospital decided to establish a neonatal health and education unit, drawing from existing nursing staff in the obstetrics and paediatric services. The structural composition of the new unit (its hierarchical organization and the roles to be played by each member) would probably be predetermined by the nursing and hospital management. A group of individuals new to each other, at least within the context of the newly established unit, would come together for the first time not only with expectations arising from the set, structural organization of the group, but also with their own unique expectations and values, goals, preconceptions, prejudices and patterns of action. This stage would be characterized by professional and interpersonal exploration, testing and exploitation of role ambiguities, a similar testing of the hierarchical strength of the group, cautious interactions with other group members, perhaps excessive interpersonal politeness, a certain rigidity of functioning, and a familiarization in the broadest sense with the group composition.

As the formal structure of the group and its membership becomes consolidated, individuals within the group may allow their own values, goals, preconceptions, prejudices and patterns of action to become more open, particularly when these conflicted with the objectives and activities of others in the group or with the objectives and activities imposed by the organization. Tacit objectives, as well as explicit ones, may emerge from group members, and those particularly wishing to exert dominance over the group may vie for positions of power and authority (often outside the formal, hierarchical structure), seeking to establish and maintain informal alliances at the expense of the existing structure. Open conflict may occur and the organization may need to re-impose its authority in order to restore functional equilibrium to the unit. This restoration (the end of storming) comes about when the functional demands of the group, the provision of a nursing service to mothers and their newborn babies, overrides the individual agendas of group members, whether these are based on real conflicts of opinion regarding the best way to provide the service or the need to exert and exploit personal power. When this happens, the group begins to function as an integrated unit, directing its collective activities towards a common goal and using the specific skills of individual members according to predetermined or emerging needs. Having achieved this functional integrity, group members may then begin to appreciate each other as individuals, to work more efficiently together and to interact socially as well as professionally.

Of course, some groups do not continue past the storming stage. While there is a recognized set of stages in group development, there is no guarantee that each of these will be successfully negotiated (just as Freud recognized developmental impasses in his system of personality development). Some groups members, having joined the group to fill some predetermined role, will have expectations and behaviours at odds with those of the group's function or with those of other group members. These people will always be disruptive to formal groups, making them difficult to operate and at times leading to their complete disintegration. Identification of disruptive members and their sensitive but rapid removal from groups usually solves this often difficult and upsetting situation.

Informal Groups

The establishment of primary/informal groups is much less structured than secondary/formal groups and is more likely to occur spontaneously. Individuals who interact frequently often develop an identification with each other over time, and are likely to form informal groups either in response to some goal-directed need or for the simple reason that they enjoy being together. As certain members leave the group, other members are likely to join. While informal groups generally do not have formal leadership, issues of power and status are likely to be just as important in these as in secondary/formal groups.

Group Norms and Cohesiveness

One of the defining characteristics of both formal and informal groups is the establishment of norms. *Group norms* are sets of behavioural expectations the group holds for all its members, in contrast to *group roles*, which refer to behavioural expectations the group holds for specific individuals (Trenholm & Jensen, 1988). More formally, a group norm is a behaviour that is expected by the group of all members within it. Norms are often also referred to as 'rules' or 'standards' of behaviour that apply to group members and are demanded by virtue of group membership (Schermerhorn *et al.*, 1985). Mere membership of that large group we know as *nurses* carries with it group norms, standards, expectations or adherence to rules. Nurses are expected to be caring, competent, ethical, compassionate, compliant, hard working and committed, and departure from these group norms may easily result in (at least *de facto*) exclusion from the group.

Without norms a group has no identity, no way of distinguishing itself from all other groups, and it has no way of governing the behaviour of the whole group. It is important to recognize that not all group norms are to the advantage of the organizations within which they operate. A group can, for example, develop norms for low work productivity (Trenholm & Jensen, 1988), which effectively restricts task output and works to the general detriment of the organization (Schermerhorn *et al.*, 1985). Nurses may, as a group, collectively impose upon themselves all of the admirable attributes we have listed above, and they are richly deserved, but in the midst of an industrial campaign, when 'work to rule' is added to these attributes, the organization becomes a formidable opponent.

In the case of formal groups, norms are usually clearly stated and known to their members. Norms for informal groups, on the other hand, are often unstated or unrecognized and, interestingly, are usually taken more seriously than those characterizing formal groups (Smither, 1988). Why this is so is not completely understood, but it is likely to relate to the difference between individual expression or choice and compliance with authority; the former is undertaken willingly but the latter only occurs in response to occupational need.

Communication is the key to establishing good norms within groups, and in maintaining them or changing outdated ones (Deaux & Wrightsman, 1988). In effective groups, members tend to talk to one another about the standards they will follow, and to reinforce each other for performing well. Indeed, the job satisfaction levels of some individuals has been related to their working with colleagues who express positive attitudes about their jobs (O'Reilly & Caldwell, in Trenholm & Jensen, 1988). Most groups have identifiable key members who are most influential, by way of their interactions with other members, in changing the norms of a particular group. A good group leader will identify these members and seek them out when there is a need to change the internal standards of a group, a point we will return to later when discussing the characteristics of group leaders.

Group norms vary in the degree to which they are accepted and adhered to by group members. Conformity to group norms is strongly influenced by a group's *cohesiveness*. While roles and norms are necessary for effective group functioning, cohesiveness makes group life enjoyable and fulfilling, providing group members with a sense of belonging (Trenholm & Jensen, 1988). Group cohesiveness has been defined as the degree to which members are attracted to a group, and motivated to remain part of that group. Members of a highly cohesive group value their membership of the group and strive to maintain positive relationships with other group members (Schermerhorn *et al.*, 1985).

The degree of group cohesiveness is affected by a range of factors including group size, homogeneity of members' characteristics, stability of membership, and agreement about the relative status of each member within the group (Wexley & Yukl, 1984). Members of highly cohesive groups, whether primary or secondary, are concerned about their group's activities and achievements. They tend, by contrast to those in less cohesive groups, to be more energetic when working on group activities, less likely to be absent from group activities, happy about performance successes within the group, and sad about its failures. Cohesive groups generally have stable memberships and foster feelings of loyalty, security and high self-esteem among their members. They satisfy a broad range of individual needs and, in short, are considered to be good for their members (Schermerhorn *et al.*, 1985).

Fostering Group Norms and Facilitating Cohesiveness

Psychological research has identified a number of norms which are fostered in groups as a way of achieving group effectiveness and cohesiveness (see Corey & Corey, 1987). Though much of this evidence has been derived from research into and evaluation of therapeutic groups of some kind or another, that is, groups designed to promote self-actualization or assist in the treatment of some psychological disorders, the general principles are broadly relevant to the operation of many kinds of groups. To facilitate group cohesiveness and maximize the effectiveness of groups to carry out their allotted purpose, group members are, for example, usually expected to:

1. attend group meetings or activities regularly and demonstrate punctuality in attendance;
2. be prepared to reveal and share personal aspects of themselves, in general becoming active participants and open contributors to group activities;

3. give honest and constructive feedback to one another regarding behaviour within the group and, if relevant, outside of the group setting;

4. focus on personal feelings and expression of these feelings within the group setting, rather than simply presenting and discussing problems in a detached and intellectualized way;

5. focus on immediate or present interactions within the group rather than on generalizations from the past or expectations of the future. Immediacy refers to the capacity of an individual to be genuine in relationships with other group members. In so far as this relates to group functioning, there is an emphasis on expression and exploration of conflicts within the group setting;

6. freely bring personal problems and concerns into the group to be discussed;

7. provide therapeutic support to one another within the group setting. Ideally, this support should help both an individual's work within the group and the processes of group functioning, rather than distracting group members from self-exploration;

8. challenge other group members to look at themselves, their behaviours, attitudes and feelings constructively and with honesty. Confrontation is the process sometimes used by members in groups to facilitate this, by expressing in a direct and caring manner a challenge for another member to examine some externally noted discrepancy between what is being said and the accompanying behaviours (compare this to the problems of mixed messages which we discussed in Chapter 6 on communication); and

9. listen to one another empathically and really hear what others say in the group context, seriously considering the messages which others send and share. (Corey & Corey, 1987)

Group norms are essentially determined by the collective will of group members. You will recall the various stages of group formation we discussed above. In the forming and storming stages, norms relating to membership issues such as expected attendance and levels of commitment are important. By the time a group reaches the performing or total integration stage, growth oriented norms relating to adaptability and change become more relevant. Irrespective of the stage of group development, however, it is important to build *positive norms* for group functioning if the group is to be effective in its activities and goals.

In the process of building positive norms, the power and importance of the group leader, whether formally chosen and appointed, or emerging from within the group by dint of prominence and influence, should not be underestimated. Schermerhorn *et al.* (1985) have identified the characteristics of group leaders (or others seeking to play a prominent and major role in a group) which have been shown to contribute significantly to the formation of positive norms. These group members must be able to:

1. act as positive role models for other group members;
2. reinforce desired behaviours in other group members;
3. control group outcomes and results by performance reviews and regular feedback to members;
4. train, orientate and encourage new group members to adopt behaviours seen as desirable for group effectiveness and performance;
5. actively recruit and select new group members who exhibit these desired group behaviours;
6. hold regular group meetings to discuss group progress, ways of improving task performance and member satisfaction; and
7. use established and appropriate group decision-making methods to reach agreement on appropriate behaviours.

Group *cohesiveness* can be also developed, maintained and increased in a number of ways. The nature of interactions between group members (group behaviour or group dynamics, in other words) can be seen to contribute to this process in important ways. Corey & Corey (1987), having reviewed the available research evidence to reveal the central features of this process, suggest that in order to bring about group cohesiveness effectively, group members must:

1. develop trust between each other by openly expressing (sharing, in other words) their personal feelings and concerns;
2. share meaningful aspects of themselves, learning to take risks with personal revelation;
3. jointly determine group and individual goals within the group, avoiding the imposition of goals satisfying only a single individual or subgroup;
4. become active, rather than passive, participants in all group activities;
5. share the leadership role within the group;
6. learn to recognize sources of conflict and deal openly with these when they arise;
7. seek to increase the attractiveness of the group to its present and potential members by dealing with matters of general interest and showing respect for all feelings and opinions expressed by group members; and
8. disclose to other group members all ideas, feelings and reactions to what occurs within the group.

There is now a great deal of evidence to suggest that members of highly cohesive groups typically experience satisfaction from group membership and affiliation. The behaviours and interactions of group members at large are clearly important in bringing this about. However, as with the establishment of positive group norms, the power and influence of group leaders is critical in bringing about group cohesiveness, and their achievement must be given real recognition. Schermerhorn *et al.* (1985) have examined those activities of group leaders which have been shown to build cohesiveness in groups. On the basis of this, they have listed a set of suggestions for group leaders concerned with the establishment of group cohesiveness. Their suggestions include:

1. inducing agreement among group members on group goals (so reducing the potential for conflict and fragmentation of group activities);
2. increasing membership homogeneity within groups (so minimizing possible sources of disagreement);
3. increasing interactions among group members (so facilitating personal relationships and commitments within groups);
4. decreasing group size (so further maximizing member homogeneity and potential for agreement);
5. introducing competition with other groups (so maximizing dissonance between groups and promoting commitment to the 'home' group and to its members);
6. allocating rewards to the group rather than to individual members (so consolidating a sense of group identity); and
7. providing physical isolation from other groups (so reducing the risk of contamination or desertion).

It is clear from the available evidence that groups work best for their members if they have positive group norms and cohesiveness, facilitated where possible by sensitive and effective group leaders. There are times, however, as we have indicated earlier, when occupational groups may in fact develop norms more consistent with low work productivity than with occupational efficiency, thus working to the detriment of the employing organization. In such instances, the group may be at odds with the organization which brought it into being, established the reasons and conditions for its continuation, and held (and continues to hold) expectations of its goals and outcomes. Under these circumstances, the rules for facilitation of group functioning may, of course, be used to counter the actions of a group which has 'left the fold' to follow an independent course. Organizations may, if they are able to infiltrate the group with influential and prominent new members, or persuade existing members to change, act to increase the formation of positive norms and cohesiveness, essentially by contriving a reversal of the activities set out above. What can be used so well to construct can, with equal effectiveness, be used to destroy if employed in a contrary manner.

Decision Making in Groups

One of the key activities in which group members engage is to make decisions, about the direction the group might take, the nature and acceptability of activities undertaken by certain group members or, indeed, the very continuation of the group itself. Schein (in Schermerhorn *et al.*, 1985), examining the processes of group decision making, found that groups use a number of different though not necessarily unrelated strategies to arrive at decisions. These strategies are discussed below.

Decision by Lack of Response
Ideas are suggested without any discussion taking place and the decision by a group to accept an idea occurs without any critical evaluation of the ideas presented. All nurses in a hospital (a group, in other words, albeit large) might, for example, be asked to offer written suggestions for the colour scheme in the new children's ward. No one replies, and the decision is made on the basis of what paint colour will be least expensive. In this sense, the decision-making process is almost a *de facto* one, with consensus being assumed simply by the absence of overt disagreement. It may reflect time pressure (and a resultant inability to devote time to the decision process), a lack of commitment to the group, a lack of commitment to the object of the decision or a belief that the decision-making process is a formality only. Whatever the cause, decision-making by lack of response in groups is relatively common.

Decision by Authority Rule
An authority figure (for example, the charge nurse on the ward) makes decisions for the group. This can be done either with or without group discussion, and has the advantage of being highly time efficient. It has the disadvantage of incurring hostility and resentment among those not involved in the decision making but expected to carry out the substance of decisions once they are made (more junior nursing staff, perhaps). Whether the decision is a good one depends on the information available to the authority figure and how well this approach is accepted by other group members. Decision by authority rule may reflect the perceived importance of the decision but may also reflect the rigidity of the organization within which decisions are being made. This approach to decision making is very individual oriented and may be used when group consensus or unanimity is unlikely to be achieved.

Decision by Minority Rule
A small number of group members are able to dominate the group and coerce it into making a decision which that small number favours. This is often done by providing a suggested decision, sometimes deceptively or inadequately documented or phrased, and then forcing quick agreement by challenging the group with the statement 'well, if no one has a problem, we will go down that path'. Once more, this approach to group decision making is likely to used when it is considered too difficult to get consensus or unanimity among group members, or when there is concern that a group decision considered important to the dominant minority might go against it if too much opportunity is provided for general consideration by the group. A small but dominant group of nurses

committed, for example, to the virtues of birthing centres might present the results of a highly favourable community survey on the need for such centres and not the medical or economic evidence on their benefits. Then, taking advantage of the immediate impression of the survey results, this small group might bring on a premature vote among their less committed colleagues as to whether the hospital should develop birthing centres rather than, say, a neonatal intensive care unit.

Decision by Majority Rule
Groups can make decisions by first finding the majority viewpoint, often through a process of voting, and then using that evidence of majority agreement as the basis for a final decision. This approach has the disadvantage of labelling individuals as 'winners' and 'losers'. The losers (the minority) may feel as though they have not had a fair say in the final decision, and may therefore harbour resentment towards the remainder (the majority) of the group. This can make the implementation of a decision difficult since support for it is fragmented, and compliance with its implementation may be less than enthusiastic. Using this approach to group decision making may possibly be due to a perceived difficulty in managing the group process so as to actually achieve complete consensus or unanimity. It is a commonly used strategy, perhaps representing a compromise but coming close to achieving real satisfaction with decision making across the group.

Decision by Consensus
Schein defines this as a state of affairs where a clear decision emerges which has the support of most group members, and even those who oppose it both feel and concede that they have been listened to and have been given a fair chance to influence the decision outcome. Consensus, therefore, does not require unanimity. Success in achieving consensus requires discipline and support from everyone in the group and a willingness to participate in the decision process and accept the outcome. Breakdowns can and do occur, however; a single, dissatisfied group member may easily destroy group consensus by vocal disagreement with a group decision. As a result, there are both potential assets and liabilities to this form of group decision making.

Decision by Unanimity
All group members agree on the course of action to be taken. Schein considers this to be a 'logically perfect' group decision method that is extremely difficult to attain in actual practice. Unanimity is rarely achieved in groups except where the outcome of the decision is likely to have an identical effect on all group members. Try to recall when you last encountered disagreement in a group meeting to consider whether or not to request a pay rise.

Decisions may, therefore, be made, in a variety of ways, each varying in the extent of group involvement. The efficiency of decision-making strategies clearly varies with the nature of the decision to be made, whether it is simple or complex, political or neutral, central or peripheral, enduring or transient and so on. Decision-making efficiency is reflected both in the process by which decisions are made, and in the outcomes that follow, as is the satisfaction which individual group members have with decisions which have been made. The research into decision making, however, clearly points to the view that decisions which fully involve all group members in the process offer several distinct advantages. Smither (1988) and Schermerhorn *et al.* (1985), having carefully examined this evidence, suggest that this occurs for a number of reasons, concerned with the following:

1. Efficiency — groups are often more efficient decision-making units than individuals, especially when large amounts of information need to be analysed in order to arrive at a decision.
2. Information processing volume — groups increase the volume of information that can be brought to bear on a problem relative to decisions made by individuals alone.
3. Understanding, acceptance and commitment — group decisions increase the degree of understanding, acceptance and commitment to the final decision, and increase the sense of responsibility among group members which is necessary to make the agreed course of action work.
4. Testing decisions — groups offer opportunities to test decisions before implementation. Group members may all offer alternative or competing solutions to a problem, so raising a full consideration of the relative merits of particular solutions, identifying potential difficulties with implementation of decisions, and raising objections where real concerns are felt. The availability of a number of perspectives arising from group consideration of decisions ensures that the 'tunnel vision' of a single perspective is avoided.

By contrast, however, as these same authors have also pointed out, the involvement of all group members in the decision-making process also has recognized disadvantages, which may take the form of:

1. Time costs — group decisions are often time consuming (for example, stopping work in order to hold discussions can have serious effects on productivity) as decision making in groups may require more time than members can spare.
2. Dubious efficiency — involving all group members is no guarantee of a superior group decision. A single, well qualified decision maker will certainly perform better than a group of inexperienced decision makers.
3. Doubtful quality — involving group members may increase the

quantity of information able to be processed, and of subsequent group decisions, but it does not necessarily improve the quality of those decisions.

4. Prematurity — involving group members in a decision process can lead those members to agree prematurely to poor decisions, particularly if pressure exists to do so.

Groupthink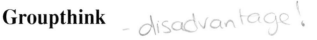

There are times when psychological factors seen to be operating within groups may inappropriately influence group decision making. When a group becomes too cohesive, for example, there is a tendency among group members to try to maintain group relations at all costs, including a decrease in the quality of decisions the group makes. The result of this influence is a phenomenon known as *groupthink*. Groupthink has been variously defined as:

1. 'A mode of thinking that people engage in when they are deeply involved in a cohesive in-group, when the members' strivings for unanimity override their motivation to realistically appraise alternative courses of action' (Janis, in Deaux & Wrightsman, 1988, p. 420).
2. 'A situation in which the social concerns of a group out-weigh concerns about quality of decision' (Janis, in Smither, 1988, p. 375).
3. 'A tendency to seek concurrence' (Longley & Pruitt, in Deaux & Wightsman, 1988, p. 420).
4. 'A tendency for highly cohesive groups to lose their critical evaluative capabilities' (Schermerhorn *et al.*, 1985, p. 336).

When group members choose to maintain the harmony of the group, and to suppress dissent in preference to expressing doubts about a forthcoming or required decision, poor decisions may result (Janis, in Baron, 1984). In this situation, critical thinking is sacrificed in order to promote group agreement and to maintain harmonious relations between group members (Trenholm & Jensen, 1988). The clear consequence of this is a trade-off, where the quality of decisions, and the potential advantages of this both for the group and for its members, are given a lower priority than the more immediate concerns of group harmony, conflict minimization, and the preservation of 'pleasant' relationships between all group members.

Janis (see also Schermerhorn *et al.*, 1985) considers group cohesion to be a key determinant in such situations. He has further argued that the basis upon which a group's cohesiveness is founded may complicate this association somewhat, suggesting that groupthink is less likely to occur in situations where the group's cohesiveness results from a base of broadly competent and demonstrably effective functioning than when it is based simply on the maintenance of a harmonious, interpersonally satisfying and conflict-free atmosphere.

It is easy to see how many kinds of groups, including groups of nurses, might engage in groupthink to the detriment of effective and efficient group activities and decisions. A small number of nurses operating within a larger group may, for example, choose against their 'better professional judgements' to adopt a clinical practice they disagree with, rather than to put the solidarity of the larger group in jeopardy by questioning the value of this practice. There is ongoing debate in clinical practice about whether terminally ill patients in pain should receive analgesic medication on demand, or whether this should be restricted to controlled doses prescribed by the physician. Groupthink could operate to influence decisions on either side of this (essentially insoluble) argument, with conformity to one side or the other occurring not because of merit but to maintain harmony within the group and, by implication, to maintain good working relationships with colleagues.

As we have outlined above, groupthink can occur in any group, whatever its structure, composition or purpose. There are, however, some steps which may be taken to minimize its influence on the process of decision making. A distillation of the evidence on this (Deaux & Wrightsman, 1988; Schermerhorn *et al.*, 1985; Smither, 1988) would suggest some combination of the following individual steps to be of potential use in restricting the occurrence and influence of groupthink. Groups should consider:

1. having all critical decisions made individually, then holding group meetings to compare the range of offered solutions;
2. openly and seriously assigning the role of critical evaluator to each group member, thereby encouraging dissidence and the sharing of objections between group members;
3. inviting outsiders to group meetings to reduce feelings of group cohesion;
4. reinforcing group members who voice criticism of a favoured plan, for their individuality, creativity and contribution;
5. creating subgroups operating under different leaders but working on the same problem;
6. avoiding partiality to one course of action, specifically by restraining a group leader from presenting a favoured plan at the outset of the discussion;
7. listing both the good and bad points of each idea as they are raised for consideration in the group;
8. having group members discuss issues with subordinates, and having done so, reporting back on the outcomes of these discussions;
9. appointing a single group member to take a purely opposing view of any favoured decision (adopt a 'devil's advocate' role) at each group meeting;

10. writing alternative scenarios for the decision process for the intentions of competing groups; and

11. holding follow-up (second chance) meetings, even after consensus is apparently achieved, on key issues where it is possible that individuals may change their minds.

While the application of all of these steps or strategies may represent overkill, their intelligent use can avoid the obvious difficulties of groupthink where this is believed to be unduly influencing decision making within groups. Above all, it is crucial for those charged with organizing groups for whatever purpose, or for taking the responsibility of leading groups towards free, rational and effective decision outcomes in the most efficient way possible, to be vigilant for the operation of groupthink and to take appropriate steps to reduce this if it is perceived to be a major difficulty. Groupthink may be no more than an inconvenient nuisance when a group of friends decide what movie they will see; it may be a severe hindrance to effective clinical practice if it prevents health professionals such as nurses from canvassing within themselves and within the groups they are members of to find all the possibilities available for effective and caring patient management.

Applications to the Practice of Nursing

Within the occupational setting there are a number of aspects and applications of group theory and practice which can be used both to enhance the performance of groups of which we are members and groups which we might lead. Within the nursing context, the *therapeutic group* is particularly important to the operations of both work-based and patient-based approaches to group activities. The term therapeutic group is a general term which indicates any of a number of related types of groups such as group counselling (or psychotherapy), self-help groups, personal growth groups, and T-groups. Therapeutic does not, in this instance, refer specifically to treating emotional and behavioural disorders, but rather to increasing people's awareness of themselves and others, assisting people to recognize the changes they want to make in their lives, and giving them some practical suggestions for bringing about these changes (Corey & Corey, 1987).

In terms of managing people (our colleagues or patients) within the nursing context, it is essential that the organizational structure (that is, nature of roles, small group behaviour, decision-making processes) as well as the needs of other individuals (that is, motivation, need for support, potential for psychological growth) are understood. Handy (in Cooper & Makin, 1984) has argued that a manager in any workplace often acts as a general medical practitioner, in that he or she is often the first person to whom others with problems will turn (the first person, for example, to whom a subordinate in trouble will turn). The process of deciding how to help a colleague or a patient in the nursing context is similar both in form and objective to this view of the manager's role as a general practitioner, in that (1) the symptoms characterizing the situation must be identified, (2) the cause of the trouble must be diagnosed, (3) a decision on how to deal with the problem has to be made, and (4) the treatment or plan of action must be created and implemented.

There are a number of types or styles of therapeutic groups which have substantial potential application to the practice of nursing. Three types of therapeutic group in particular will be considered below, two with potential direct application for patient groups (group therapy and group counselling) and the other with potential application to work-based or occupational groups of colleagues (sensitivity-training groups).

Group versus Individual Therapies

The basic objectives of group counselling and individual treatment programs are similar. Both seek to help clients achieve self-direction, integration, self-responsibility, self-acceptance and an understanding of their motivations and patterns of behaviour. In both cases, the counsellor (whether nurse or other helping professional) needs the characteristics and skills which we have outlined in Chapter 2. There are, however, important differences between individual and group counselling (Hopson, in Cooper & Makin, 1984, p. 275), these being that:

1. Effective group counselling requires an understanding of group dynamics whereas individual work, for obvious reasons, does not.
2. The counselling or therapeutic group situation provides good opportunities to try out different ways of relating to and experiencing psychological and personal intimacy with other people. The physical and psychological closeness of participants in group settings can be emotionally rewarding and supportive for all involved. All participants in therapeutic groups are given a first hand opportunity to test others' perceptions of themselves, whereas this is limited only to the patient and therapist in individual work.
3. Participants in counselling or therapeutic groups not only receive help themselves from their involvement with the group, but they also help one another. Through group counselling, helping skills are generated by a larger group of people than is possible in individual counselling.
4. Participants in counselling or therapeutic groups often discover that other people have similar problems to their own, thus setting individual concerns into a broader context, perhaps even one of normality, and providing the emotional comfort which accompanies this realization.

5. Participants in counselling or therapeutic groups learn to make effective use of other people as helping agents. Moreover, as group participants learn to cope with their individual problems, and distance themselves from reliance on the group, levels of self-esteem increase, usually accompanied by broad improvements in psychological state.

Group Therapy

Many people are advised to participate in group therapy because a specific psychological disorder such as depression, anxiety or a psychosomatic illness of some kind has been diagnosed by a health professional, and he or she feels that group treatment will provide the most effective means of alleviating the disorder. Some therapy groups are specifically oriented in their content and organization towards the treatment of particular disorders; groups for depression, social skilfulness, assertiveness and the like are examples of this. Others take a more general approach, operating on the assumption that interpersonal exchange within a group setting consisting largely of people with psychological problems will ultimately work for the better. The former groups tend to be highly structured, closed ended, short in duration and have well defined objectives. The latter are far less well defined, directing broad attention to past experiences, personality and to a range of inferred but unconscious factors, allowing a relatively unfocused interchange between a diverse range of people with problems.

Nurses working particularly (but of course, not exclusively) within psychiatric hospital settings may be called upon to conduct group therapy along the lines of either (or both) of these two models. Nurses may act as co-therapists with other mental health professionals (psychiatrists, clinical psychologists and the like) or, increasingly, as group therapists in their own right, taking complete responsibility for the organization and running of therapeutic groups. The roles and tasks of the nurse as a group therapy leader will be considered later in this chapter. In general terms, however, the conduct and effectiveness of group therapy is based on a number of assumptions about the functions of groups and of the participants in them. These are:

1. Every person (whether patient or otherwise) has the potential to make decisions conducive to their own psychological and emotional growth through increased self-awareness, stopping old and maladaptive behaviours, and practising new behaviours.
2. Every person has a drive to seek information on his or her self and how he or she interacts with others, from awareness of his or her own psychological, emotional and physical dimensions.
3. Within a group, each person has an opportunity to achieve the goals

of therapy, that is, increased self-awareness, stopping old and maladaptive behaviours and practising new behaviours. For this to occur, the negative consequences of openly expressing oneself within the group setting need to be eliminated, and patients must be provided with a role model (often the group leader) to pattern themselves after.

Naar (1982) has set out the ideal nature and sequence of events which are expected to occur in effective therapeutic groups. In his analysis, these are that:

1. each group member should accept that the rules of group functioning act to eliminate the possibly negative consequences of participants openly expressing themselves;
2. each group member should be prepared to give some feedback to other group members, such that when this communication is genuine, the feedback is positive;
3. each group member should encourage other group members to use the group setting to seek increased awareness of and deal with unresolved conflicts, even though this may lead to feelings of distress;
4. each group member may experience stress and this may elicit feelings of sympathy, affection and support for their problems from the rest of the group;
5. each group member should gradually accept the exposed real self of each other member, resulting in increased self-acceptance and decreased defensiveness in everybody; and
6. each group member should discard unrealistic coping mechanisms, thereby liberating energy that may be used more constructively.

While Naar does not present these stages as either necessary or sufficient conditions for the achievement of positive individual change within the setting of a therapeutic group, it is clear that if these conditions are satisfied this greatly enhances the chances of both efficient and effective therapeutic group functioning, and positive psychological changes for individual participants in the therapeutic group.

Group Counselling

The counselling group, like the therapeutic group, usually focuses on a particular type of personal or social problem, though its focus is typically broader and the group participants are typically at a higher level of coping than individuals specifically diagnosed as psychiatrically impaired. As such, group counselling is often carried out in non-residential medical settings, such as community mental health clinics, outpatient hospital services, school- or university-based counselling centres and occupational environments. Since nurses play important roles in many of these settings, they are often involved in running counselling groups. The general orientation of counselling groups is toward the resolution of specific, relatively short term issues rather than deeply ingrained, chronic psychological disorder.

Group counselling has both preventive and remedial aims. The group involves an interpersonal process that focuses on conscious thoughts, feelings and behaviours. It is characterized by an orientation towards emotional and psychological growth, with an emphasis on discovering inner resources of personal strength by helping members, through the group, to deal constructively with barriers preventing optimal development. As Corey & Corey (1987) have told us, counselling groups provide the support and the challenge necessary for honest self-exploration. The focus of a counselling group is most often determined by the members themselves. People involved in group counselling tend to be largely well functioning individuals free of conspicuous psychiatric symptoms and obvious maladaptations. They do not require extensive personality change and their problems relate either to dealing more effectively with routine (though possibly severe) life changes or to finding means to cope with the stresses of continual or unique situational crises (Corey & Corey, 1987). For example, patients faced with a severe or life threatening illness may often benefit from short term participation in counselling groups to reinforce already existing coping strategies and to resolve specific anxieties regarding their own illness within a context of sharing with others facing the same crisis. Women or men facing the breakup of a long term relationship (the threat of divorce, perhaps) may also find help in a counselling group where fears, frustrations, anger, uncertainty and grief, all associated with the breakup of the relationship, may be shared, discussed and resolved. Parents of terminally ill children often use counselling groups to share with each other the concerns of the present and the threatened grief of the future, in a setting of mutual understanding and trust. The amount of clinical and research literature on group counselling is large; examples are abundant and there is clear evidence that group counselling benefits those not formally psychiatrically ill but still facing some personal crisis and in distress because of it. In many instances, nurses will be immediate observers of such crises and, indeed, they will often be participants in the complex situations surrounding these. The nurse's skills as a group counsellor, whether her role is a formal one (as a designated leader of a formally constituted group) or an informal one (as, for example, a clinically involved and professional participant in an informal group coming together around a seriously ill or dying patient), will therefore be in almost constant demand.

T-groups or Interpersonal Skills Training

T- (or training) groups, sometimes called interpersonal skills training groups, tend to emphasize the human relations skills required to function successfully in an organization. Nurses may find themselves either involved in or expected to run such groups within the workplace. In these groups the emphasis is on training through experience, and in a psychologically 'open' environment in which experimentation is possible, new ideas are encouraged, information can be collected and analysed, and decisions can be made or problems solved. Frequently, these groups are task oriented and the focus is on specific organizational problems, such as 'how can nurses express themselves more creatively in the clinical situation?' or 'how can different members of the health professions work harmoniously and effectively together in the occupational context?' (Corey & Corey, 1987).

In some cases, an individual's performance can be noticeably hindered by problems among members of work groups. Productivity may be hampered, for example, because members of different professional groups refuse to cooperate with one another in crucial and interactive professional tasks, or communication may be disrupted by rivalries when the staffs of two hospitals are forced to merge. In such instances, T-groups may prove useful in helping to solve emerging problems (Smither, 1988, p. 376). The focus of T-groups is on the group process of interaction and communication rather than on personal growth for individual participants (Corey & Corey, 1987). Thus, T-groups attempt to increase the awareness among group members of the psychological factors that may adversely affect communication within the group and, by implication, the occupational task (Smither, 1988).

T- or interpersonal skills groups start with the assumption that individuals will interact as they typically would in the workplace in the group meeting. That is, those who are generally assertive will try to dominate the meeting, just as those who are more timid will be hesitant about participating in the group discussions. One of the purposes of a T-group meeting is to identify patterns or styles of group interaction among participants, with the assumption that such identification is likely to lead to insights about how those same individuals are being perceived by their colleagues in the occupational setting (Smither, 1988). In the group setting, participants are free to explore their feelings about each other and about the ways in which relationships with colleagues can be improved both in and outside of the group. Participants are encouraged not to be hostile or defensive in their interactions with others, but to listen carefully to what others are saying. Advocates of this method believe that this openness in communication within the T-group setting will result in improved relations between group members once they return, as colleagues, to the occupational environment (Smither, 1988).

The role of the leader of a T- or interpersonal skills group is not to direct the group but to conduct the group and its interactions in such a way as to provide a model of correct and appropriate group behaviour. The leader encourages group members to share their feelings, to keep their focus on the communication processes that are occurring in the meeting, and to maintain confidentiality about group activities after the meeting is over. The leader must also assure participants that what transpires during the group meeting will not threaten the job or security of any participant (Smither, 1988). Without this, trust in the group and its leader, and confidence in the certainty and usefulness of its outcome, may be diminished to a point where the group will not be able to achieve the desired goals. The importance of effective group leadership in this, as in other groups so far discussed in this chapter, cannot therefore be underestimated.

Effective Group Leadership

The role of the group counsellor or (in the case of non-therapeutic groups) the group leader is to structure the activities of the group, to see that a climate favourable to productive work is maintained, to facilitate participant interaction and to encourage group members to translate their insights into concrete plans of action for personal change. To a large extent, group leaders carry out this role by teaching group members to focus on the present and to establish personal goals that will provide direction for the group as a whole (Corey & Corey, 1987).

Effective group leadership is contingent not only on the personal characteristics of the group leader but also on the basic counselling or leadership skills which individuals bring to particular group situations. Corey & Corey (1987, pp. 14–27) have provided a comprehensive overview of these *personal characteristics* and *group leadership skills*, and in their view, if group leaders are to be effective in their tasks, they should possess at least a large proportion of these characteristics.

More specifically, the effective group leader should possess *personal characteristics* which show:

1. a willingness in group situations to be vulnerable, to confront both themselves and others, to act on beliefs, to examine their inner selves, to be honest, and to openly express their fears within the group setting;
2. a willingness to teach by example and to talk openly about their feelings at appropriate times;
3. an ability to be emotionally present, to be touched by another person's distress and joy, to experience emotions fully, and to be compassionate and empathic;
4. an interest in the welfare of others, by showing respect, trust and valuing of others;

5. a belief and trust in the value of what they are doing;
6. a willingness to be open with oneself, with others, to new experiences, and to different lifestyles, attitudes and values;
7. an ability to deal frankly with personal criticism and with criticism of other group members;
8. an ability to know who one personally 'is' (personal self-awareness) and what one wants to achieve, both within the group and more broadly;
9. an ability to withstand pressure emerging from within the group and to remain vitalized in spite of this;
10. a willingness to identify ways to seek new experiences and to draw on one's own emotions;
11. an awareness of one's personal needs and motivations;
12. an enjoyment of humour and an ability to laugh at one's own human frailties; and
13. the capacity to be spontaneously creative, involving both the ability to detect clues from within group interactions and to create new ways of exploring group problems. (Corey & Corey, 1987, pp. 14–27)

Group effectiveness is also dependent on *group leadership skills*, that is, specific strategies and techniques as opposed to strictly personal characteristics, and the effective group leader should show a well developed ability:

1. to listen to others as they communicate, absorbing the content of the messages, noting gestures and subtle changes in voice or expression, and sensing underlying meanings to communications;
2. to convey through feedback the essence of what a group member has communicated so that the person can more fully understand his or her own message and appreciate that it has been understood and respected by a significant other;
3. to focus on key underlying issues in group communications and be able to clarify confusing or conflicting feelings, both at the group and the individual level;
4. to be caring and open in the group setting, and display a well developed ability to discern subtle, non-verbal messages as well as those messages transmitted more directly from one individual to another;
5. to offer convincing and rational explanations for certain behaviours seen to emerge within the group or symptoms evident within particular individuals and presented by them for comment and explanation;
6. to question constructively what is occurring in groups, both at the individual level and at the level of total group interaction;
7. to help open up clear channels of communication and to increase the group's collective sense of responsibility for the direction it is taking;

8. to formulate clear and concise overviews of information both presented by group members and arising from the functioning of the group itself;
9. to relate what one individual is doing or saying within the group to the concerns of another individual or of the group as a whole;
10. to deal with behaviour which may be disruptive to group functioning, and to manage discrepancies in opinion (conflict) which might come about during the operation of the group and which might lead to disruptive group behaviours;
11. to give appropriate behavioural feedback to individual group participants where it is considered that this will be of benefit to their goals of growth or change, or to the effective functioning of the group as a whole;
12. to control negative activities of group members, such as gossiping, invading another's privacy, breaking confidences and so on, particularly where this might disrupt the structure and function of the group;
13. to delineate observed behavioural problems of group members, and both choose and implement appropriate interventions within the group setting;
14. to offer a range of possible outcomes arising from alternative plans of action, and to encourage an exchange of views among group members on how realistic they consider each plan might be; and
15. to appraise the movement and direction of the group. (Corey & Corey, 1987, pp. 14–27)

It is important to remember, when considering the attributes of effective group leaders, that both personal characteristics and group leadership skills are neccessary for the task to be successfully completed. The former set of attributes are reminiscent of those we spoke about in Chapters 2 and 3, on the nurse as an effective counsellor. They are attributes which relate to the personal qualities of the individual, able to be established through training, but reflecting the unique capacities of the person to relate to another person so as to help them realize their potential more and live a more enjoyable life. These attributes presuppose a high degree of psychological integration within the group leader, a capacity for honesty and an overall approach typified by caring.

The group leadership skills are more closely akin to those we set out in Chapter 6 on communication in the practice of nursing. These are technical skills based on an understanding of the communication process and a capacity to translate this understanding into action within the dynamic and developing process that is a group. Once more, these skills are open to establishment through learning and instruction, though their application requires experience and the ability to switch quickly and skilfully from theory to action, and back again, as the group situation demands. Armed with these skills, however, nurses will be capable of leading and participating in many forms of groups including therapeutic groups, counselling groups and T- or interpersonal skills training groups. Moreover, the very nature, structure and function of nursing practice almost guarantees that she will be called upon to do so.

Summary

In this chapter an attempt has been made to define groups and delineate the features of primary and secondary groups. The stages of group development were described, as were the nature and process of group norms, cohesiveness and decision making in groups. The possible difficulties involved in group decision making were described with particular reference to the phenomenon of groupthink. Then, various applications of group theory and practice to nursing were considered. The differences between group and individual approaches to patient care were assessed and three types of therapeutic groups were then described (two with potential applications for patient groups and one with potential application for work-based groups). It was argued that irrespective of the type of group, there are a number of essential personal qualities and group leadership skills which nurses should possess in order for them to run therapeutic groups. These were outlined in detail, and presented as the first pathway to the nurse's effective participation, as leader, in the diverse range of groups which are central to nursing practice.

References/Reading List

Baron, R.S. (1984). Group dynamics. In A.S. Kahn (ed.), *Social Psychology*. Dubuque, Iowa: William C. Brown.

Bednar, R.L. & Kaul, T.J. (1985). Experiential group research: results, questions and suggestions. In S.L. Garfield & A. Bergin (eds), *Handbook for Psychotherapy and Behavior Change*. New York: John Wiley & Sons.

Bednar, R.L. & Lawlis, F. (1971). Empirical research in group psychotherapy. In A.E. Bergin & S.L. Garfield (eds), *Handbook for Psychotherapy and Behavior Change*. New York: John Wiley & Sons.

Cartwright, D. & Zander, A. (eds) (1968). *Group Dynamics: Research and Theory*. New York: Harper & Row.

Cooper C.L. & Makin, P. (eds) (1984). *Psychology for Managers*. Trowbridge, Wiltshire: Macmillan.

Corey, M.S. & Corey, G. (1987). *Groups: Process and Practice*. Monterey, California: Brooks/Cole.

Deaux, K. & Wrightsman, L.S. (1988). *Social Psychology*. Pacific Grove, California: Brooks/Cole.

Hare, A.P. (1976). *Handbook of Small Group Research*. New York: Free Press.

Hopson, B. (1984). Counselling and helping. In C.L. Cooper & P. Makin (eds) *Psychology for Managers*. Trowbridge, Wiltshire: Macmillan.

Janis, I.L. (1972). *Victims of Groupthink*. Boston: Houghton Mifflin.

Jewell, L.N. & Reitz, H.J. (1981). *Group Effectiveness in Organizations*. Glenview, Illinois: Scott, Foresman & Company.

Kaplan, H.I. & Sadock, B.J. (eds) (1983). *Comprehensive Group Psychotherapy*. Baltimore: Williams & Wilkins.

Kerr, S. (ed.) (1979). *Organizational Behavior*. New York: John Wiley & Sons.

Leavitt, H.J., Pondy, L.R. & Boje, D.M. (eds) (1980). *Readings in Managerial Psychology*. Chicago: University of Chicago Press.

Naar, R. (1982). *A Primer of Group Psychotherapy*. New York: Human Sciences Press.

Napier, R.W. & Gershenfield, M.K. (1981). *Groups: Theory and Experience*. Boston: Houghton Mifflin.

Napier, R.W. & Gershenfield, M.K. (1983). *Making Groups Work: A Guide for Group Leaders*. Boston: Houghton Mifflin.

Schermerhorn, J.R., Hunt, J.G. & Osborn, R.N. (1985). *Managing Organizational Behavior*. New York: John Wiley & Sons.

Shaw, M.E. (1976). *Group Dynamics: The Psychology of Small Group Behaviour*. New York: McGraw-Hill.

Smither, R.D. (1988). *The Psychology of Work and Human Performance*. New York: Harper & Row.

Trenholm, S. & Jensen, A. (1988). *Interpersonal Communication*. Belmont, California: Wadsworth Publishing Company.

Tuckman, B.W. (1965). Development sequences in small groups. *Psychological Bulletin*, 63, 384–399.

Wexley, K.N. & Yukl, G.A. (1984). *Organizational Behaviour and Personnel Psychology*. Homewood, Illinois: Richard D. Irwin.

9
Burnout and its Management in Nursing

No matter how it is viewed, nursing is a personally taxing profession. It carries with it a broad range of duties and responsibilities, and a complex and demanding set of both personal and professional expectations, often in the absence of anything close to adequate support and backup. Nurses are expected to be technically competent and personally caring. In addition, they are required to be dominant in some circumstances and subservient in others. They are also expected to be respectful of the organizational hierarchy within which they work even though that hierarchy may sometimes lack logic. Above all, nurses are expected to be present and available at all times to attend to the many and often conflicting needs of their patients and their superiors. Not surprisingly, burnout is a relatively common experience within the nursing profession.

What is Burnout?

Over the past two decades, there has been increased interest in the phenomenon of *burnout*. Indeed the term burnout has become very common and is a popular explanation for a whole range of personal and occupational problems. As such, it has had a major impact on assumptions and expectations regarding certain types of work. However, research into burnout is still in its infancy; the characteristics of burnout and the number and kinds of people afflicted by burnout have yet to be clearly delineated. None the less, to the extent that burnout has become legitimized and even expected of certain types of workers, particularly those in the health service professions, it may already have had a broad effect on the motivation of many in these professions to continue to work hard at their jobs. Indeed, it has been argued by some that burnout is simply an excuse for failing to do an adequate job (Farber, 1983a). Heifetz & Bersani (1983) state that there is an unquestionable and understandable attractiveness to the idea of burnout. The label 'burned out' often seems to serve as a partial remedy for the condition it describes. That is, in the absence of other evidence of professional accomplishment, burnout provides some consolation as a badge of martyred dedication and a reason for diminished performance.

It seems unfair, however, simply to dismiss burnout as a popular but insubstantial topic used only to elicit the sympathy of others. Rather, as this chapter will show, burnout is a serious and complex problem that affects the welfare of a large number of health service workers, and has the potential to affect the patients who are dependent on the services of these professionals (Farber, 1983a).

To date, there has been a lack of agreement as to what burnout actually is (Farber, 1983a). Indeed, according to Maslach, a pioneering researcher in the area, there is no single definition of burnout that has yet been accepted as a standard. None the less, some concerted effort has been made to define burnout with some technical precision. In the simplest terms, the existence of burnout has been defined as: 'when you are no longer effective and you no longer care' (Selder & Paustian, 1989, p. 73). Maslach (1976), in a somewhat more detailed comment, suggested that burnt out professionals are those who: 'lose all concern, all emotional feelings for the persons they work with and come to treat them in detached or even dehumanized ways' (p. 16). Pines & Maslach (1978) have described burnout as: 'a syndrome of physical and emotional exhaustion, involving the development of a negative self concept, negative job attitudes, and a loss of concern and feelings [by workers] for clients' (p. 223). Freudenberger (1974, 1975), the originator of the concept, has defined burnout as a state of physical and emotional depletion which results from the condition of an individual's work. More recently, Freudenberger & Richelson (1980) described burnout as: 'someone in a state of fatigue or frustration brought about by devotion to a cause, way of life, or relationship that failed to produce the expected reward' (p. 13), or a 'disease of over commitment' (in Cherniss & Krantz, 1983). In other words, when what we expect is dramatically opposed to what is, and yet we still persist in trying to fulfil that unrealistic expectation, the possibility for burning out increases.

Perhaps the most comprehensive definition of burnout is provided by Maslach who, in her (1976) work on burnout, has established the notion as a potential problem for all health professionals involved in direct patient care. Much of this early work was based on information collected from interviews with a range of health service workers (for example, physicians and social workers). From this research, a description of the burnout syndrome was derived with particular emphasis on health care professionals. Burnout was considered to relate to a loss of concern for people. More specifically, Maslach (1982) defined burnout as: 'a syndrome of emotional exhaustion, depersonalization, and reduced personal accomplishment that can occur among individuals who do "people work" of some kind' (p. 3).

Emotional exhaustion refers to the desire to withdraw from others and from work. The individual feels all used up and unable to continue in his or her normal day to day activities, totally drained and unable to see a way of becoming emotionally charged again.

Depersonalization refers to the almost dehumanized response which develops towards those around, including patients and colleagues. The afflicted person begins to distrust and even to dislike everyone, not only reacting negatively to people, but also being rude or, in extreme cases, even failing to provide an appropriate level of care for those for whom she is responsible.

Reduced personal accomplishment refers to the dissatisfaction that an individual begins to feel toward her personal and professional accomplishments, both in the occupational setting and toward herself. She begins to see herself and her abilities as totally inadequate, and begins to blame herself for everything that goes wrong.

In summary, while Maslach has expressed some real concern at the lack of a standard definition of burnout, it is quite clear that burnout refers to a negative work experience that produces a range of negative occupational and personal consequences.

Being burned out means that the total emotional, physical and psychological energy of the person has been consumed in trying to survive within the occupational setting. The consequences of trying to keep afloat in this setting also impact on the afflicted person's social, personal and family areas of activity. Burnout occurs because of a disparity between demand and supply; the demands of the occupation exceed the personal capacity of the individual to supply.

Why Address Burnout in Nursing?

Burnout was originally conceived for and investigated within the health and social services fields (Freudenberger, 1989), and the literature on burnout is primarily concerned with health service professionals (Jayaratne & Chess, 1983). A large proportion of this rapidly growing work has emphasized the causal role of excessive demands, unsatisfactory training and inadequate skills of service providers in producing burnout. Put simply, there is thought to be a significant mismatch between the demands of the occupational tasks undertaken by health service workers and the capacities of these workers to cope with such excessive or complex demands (Heifetz & Bersani, 1983).

Burnout, many will say, is endemic to nursing. Certainly, the bulk of writing and research on burnout has arisen from the often reported problems of those in the helping professions and examples of nurses experiencing professional burnout are common in the literature. Wessells *et al.* (1989) report the case of a nurse working in an outpatient muscular dystrophy clinic who had reported increasing feelings of distress in specific areas of her work. She found, for example, that it was difficult to talk to parents of children attending the clinic when she had to address the issue of impending hospitalization. She experienced helplessness and hopelessness if required to speak with emotionally distressed parents, and felt responsible for what was happening to her patients. Frustration and stress welled up in her and her work performance began to be impaired. Coronary care nurses, again in an environment where life threatening illness is faced daily, have also reported feelings of frustration and stress in their work. Wessells *et al.* singled out the example of a nurse who became extremely upset with a physician whom she felt did not adequately deal with the needs of patients. In so many instances, the emotional and physical demands of nursing have been reported to impose sufficient strain on nurses to bring about significant personal costs.

Indeed, for many nurses, there appears to be a certain inevitability about burnout. As one nurse who recently quit her job put it: 'Burnout is not the experience of having too much to do but rather it is not having the energy to do things you know you can do and not enjoying the things you used to love to do' (Selder & Paustian, 1989, p.73).

At a pragmatic level, there are three reasons why it is important to focus on burnout in nursing. First, it has now been demonstrated beyond reasonable doubt that the problem of burnout can have serious personal and occupational consequences for health service workers, and it is important to address and attempt to reduce the suffering of these people. Second, apart from the personal suffering which might be experienced by these people, from an economic perspective literally billions of dollars are lost each year as a direct consequence of their inability to function adequately in their jobs. Third, the problems which providers of health care seem to experience can also have unintended consequences for the patients they care for. The quality of health care can diminish as a consequence of burnt out practitioners (Cartwright, 1979). Indeed, institutions such as hospitals and mental health agencies have been the subject of frequent and often harsh criticism for the quality of care they provide. One of the central themes underlying much of this dissatisfaction has been that these institutions are often seen as impersonal, cold, and dehumanizing (Eisenstat & Felner, 1983). Clearly, agencies can and do differ in the quality of care they provide and this may relate to the level of burnout experienced by health care service workers in these occupational settings.

Aside from this, it has been suggested (Freudenberger & Richelson, 1980) that that segment of the population which is attracted to the helping professions (nurses form a large part of this group) is particularly sensitive to the feelings and behaviours of others. The personal qualities of health care service workers, in other words, may have induced them into this set of professions in the first place. Such people may, therefore, be more vulnerable to the empathic experience of distress and despair seen in others, and so more likely to fall victim, at some stage, to the despair which a lot of their patients bring with them. The essence of nursing (and other helping professions) is service delivery of a highly personalized nature, requiring high levels of emotional commitment. Because health service workers care about people, they are particularly sensitive to the social dimension of their work, and consequently they may be vulnerable to the dangers of burnout (Pines, 1983). The work of the helping professions is both taxing and tough. There are few rewards and there are innumerable and constant pressures. Consequently a large number of highly skilled and dedicated individuals are lost to these professions.

Part of the problem for some nurses may be that they perceive themselves to be 'ideal' caregivers; according to Selder & Paustian (1989), the *ideal caregiver personality* is characterized by the belief that an individual must work hard at all times, must be everything to everyone, must always try to help everyone, must never be wrong, must always try to improve and must sacrifice personal needs to the needs of others.

Patterson (1980) has also investigated the myths which those in the helping professions bring to their jobs, illustrated by such statements as:

1. my job is my life, which means I must spend long hours on the job and have no leisure time;
2. I must be totally competent and able to help everyone;
3. I must be liked and approved of by everyone; and
4. if I receive any negative feedback, there must be something wrong with what I do.

There are a number of problems in seeing one's self as a perfect caregiver. Failure to live up to the ideal of personal and professional perfection causes a person to doubt his or her competence, have a lower self-esteem and image, and a tendency to step away from the situation as a basic means of self-protection. Nurses, plagued by such irrational beliefs, will come to experience greater and greater perceived disparities between demand and capacity, between expected competence and personal skill and between required and available energy. They will, therefore, experience a diminution of their own image as a competent and caring health professional able to contribute to the well-being of others, and as this happens they will experience personal distress and a compelling tendency to create psychological barriers between themselves and the attributed source of their distress, that is, their work and patients. They will, in effect, experience burnout.

Along with perceiving themselves to be 'ideal' caregivers, many of those people working in the helping professions struggle with achieving what has been called 'detached concern' (Lief & Fox, in Pines, Aronson & Kafry, 1981). This is a stance in which the empathic health professional is sufficiently detached in attitudes toward the patient to be able to exercise sound medical judgement and maintain equanimity, while at the same time displaying enough concern for the patient to provide sensitive and understanding care. In this way the patient, rather than just his or her physical/psychological condition, becomes the concern of the health professional.

Detached concern is a difficult balance to achieve and harder still to maintain. On the one hand, there is the danger of becoming overly involved, and on the other hand, the danger of becoming completely detached. In the former case the professional loses objectivity and therefore the ability to help effectively, while in the latter case there is insufficient involvement to motivate the professional to help successfully. Failure to achieve the balance may easily lay the basis for burnout.

The problem of burnout, then, is well known in the profession of nursing. Quantitative studies show that it exists, and there is sufficient well reasoned theory to provide insights as to why it should exist. The economic costs, while difficult to establish precisely, are likely to be large, and the personal costs, while impossible to quantify at all, are so much in evidence in individual experience that they cannot be ignored. The study and management of burnout in nursing therefore poses an issue of considerable importance.

Antecedents of Burnout

Following largely from the issues discussed above, Pines *et al.* (1981) have identified three common antecedents of burnout in the helping professions: emotionally taxing work, humanitarian personalities, and a client-centred orientation. Let us discuss each of these in turn.

By the very nature of their jobs, those working in the human and health service professions often work in emotionally demanding situations for long periods of time. Consequently, they are exposed to the whole gambit of patient problems and, moreover, are expected to be both professionally competent and personally caring in all these situations. Nurses, as a particular professional group, are called upon to deal with the fears, anger, despair and hopelessness of their patients. They are often involved in emergency situations and regularly come face to face with patients suffering incurable diseases; they must also regularly confront death itself. There is no doubt, therefore, that nursing brings with it the performance of emotionally taxing work.

It has been found that those working in the health service professions often exhibit similar personality patterns, both as members of and before joining these professions. They tend, for example, to be sensitive, empathic, humanitarian in their beliefs and altruistic in their outlook. Nurses, as one particular group, may be seen to have these orientations to their work; essentially, they want to be in a job where they can help people in trouble. There is a tendency among nurses to see themselves as understanding, unselfish, helpful and sympathetic to others. Typically, they describe themselves as liking people and wanting to work with people. These characteristics, admirable as they are, have regrettably been shown to increase vulnerability to burnout.

Those working in the health service professions are there to provide a service to those in need. The professional's role is to provide assistance, support and understanding. However, the helping relationship is asymmetrical by nature; that is, it is a relationship in which the needs of the patient come first, so that the professional gives and the patient receives. For some nurses, there will be inherent rewards in the work they do. There is a real risk, however, that the needs of the nurse as helper will not be met by a system that, at least tacitly, expects the providers of helping relationships to inhibit actively and routinely the expression of any expectations or hopes of their own regarding their jobs.

These three antecedents of burnout are present in nearly all health service work, and make the process of burnout a highly likely one for many who choose this professional path.

Symptoms/Stages of Burnout

Burnout is a multidimensional phenomenon; it is both an individual and a societal concern. Occupational features such as high job turnover, high absenteeism and lowered work productivity may indicate burnout. Burnout may also be indicated by the presence of in a host of psychological problems ranging from personal anxiety and distress to an inability to provide an adequate service to patients, or in extreme cases, overt neglect.

In nursing it has been found that burnout has its origins in patient care issues, nurses' expectations of themselves, interstaff issues and institutional demands (Burgess, in Freudenberger, 1989). More specifically, Freudenberger, Maslach, Pines and others have argued that the basic causes of burnout lie with the disruptive emotional aspects of patient care, such as overly demanding patients, unreasonable patient behaviours, illnesses (especially those involving constant and extreme pain and suffering and/or certainty of death) that are difficult to treat and which may lead to a strong emotional response from the health service workers, as well as the recognition that there is sometimes a denial by caregivers of their emotional responses to a patient's pain. Exposure to the suffering and sometimes the death of patients has the potential to affect caregivers in such a way as to cause them to approach caring in a mechanical way. The result seems to be a continuous negative contact between the caregiver and the environment in which he or she works.

For example, Pines' work (Pines *et al.*, 1981; Pines, 1983), which involved empirical analyses of burnout data from large samples of nurses in North America, has demonstrated that burnout is significantly correlated with reduced satisfaction with work, life and oneself, as well as with poor physical health (increases in sleep disorders, headaches, loss of appetite, nervousness, backaches and stomach aches). In addition, burnout has been found to be related to hopelessness (and suicidal potential), alcoholism, tardiness and an intention to leave one's job.

Edelwich & Brodsky (in Weiner, 1989) have examined the course of the development of burnout, and have delineated four stages of disillusionment leading to the phenomenon, these being:

1. enthusiasm — the individual has unrealistic expectations of her job and makes too great a personal investment in it;
2. stagnation — the individual becomes aware of the difference between what she thought the job was and what it really is;
3. frustration — the individual feels disappointed with her job and begins to question her adequacy as a professional and her reason for staying in the job at all; and
4. apathy — the individual becomes apathetic as a defence against frustration.

To make this a little more concrete as regards the kinds of situations nurses might experience, let us consider the following. The overwhelming majority of nurses enter their profession with enthusiasm. Research evidence on occupational choice suggests that nurses are among the most initially committed to their work, displaying at the outset of their careers both idealism and energy at the prospect of working towards the health of others. There is, however, an equally abundant body of research evidence supporting the view that organizational rules and structures within the nursing environment are restrictive, rigid, sometimes apparently irrational and often seen as counteractive to the process of caring for others. Moreover, the poor financial rewards of nursing compared with many of the other helping professions nurses come into contact with in their day to day activities have, for a long time, been a source of occupational contention and dissatisfaction.

Even the normal conditions of nursing might, therefore, be seen to give rise to stagnation in the work situation. For some nurses, the rigidity of the profession and of its organization, particularly in the face of high levels of initial enthusiasm, an overriding concern for patients and their care, and an incapacity to reconcile the rigidity of the system with the perceived needs of patients, leads to the rapid development of frustration. As frustration progresses and becomes consolidated by the continued interaction of the nurse with the 'system', a self-protective detachment is seen in the form of apathy, and in a simple sequence of events it is therefore easy to conceive of the onset of burnout.

There is general consensus that the symptoms of burnout include attitudinal, behavioural, physical and interpersonal components (Gilliland & James, 1988; Farber, 1983a). Gilliland & James (1988, pp. 448–449) have produced a convenient and concise set of descriptors of burnout which, while not exhaustive, provide a good guide to many of the difficulties experienced by service delivery workers experiencing crises. These characteristics are shown in Box 9.1

The importance of occupational organizational structures in the development of burnout has not been overlooked. Farber (1983b) has set out four 'cornerstones' for burnout which might impact on the individual within the workplace. Specifically, Farber has identified problems of role ambiguity, role conflict and role overload, as well as feelings of inconsequentiality, as organizational factors which might contribute to burnout among health service workers. More specifically:

Box 9.1   *Characteristics of burnout (drawn from Gilliland & James, 1988, pp. 448–449)*

Attitudinal: affective disorder or emotional distress; boredom and depersonalization; pessimism, emptiness, cynicism and callousness; guilt and helplessness; compulsiveness, obsessiveness and a hypercritical view of others; distrust of others; sick humour directed to clients.

Behavioural: impaired work efficiency; overuse of alcohol and illicit drugs; loss of creativity, enjoyment and control; absenteeism and neglect of work; high job turnover; complaints and hyper-responsivity to stress.

Physical: psychosomatic symptoms and illness; muscle tension; fatigue, immunological vulnerability; large fluctuations in appetitive behaviours (tobacco, caffeine and food consumption); sleep disturbance; menstrual difficulties; occupational injuries; exacerbation of existing illnesses.

Interpersonal: withdrawal from others; reduction in social networks; loneliness; avoidance of interpersonal contacts; imposition of status hierarchies onto personal and client relationships; relationship breakdowns; isolation and anger; incapacity to separate professional and private lives.

1. role ambiguity refers to a lack of clarity regarding a worker's rights, responsibilities, status, goals and so on with respect to themselves or their institutions;
2. role conflict refers to the situation where inconsistent, incompatible or inappropriate demands are placed upon an individual;
3. role overload refers to having too much to do or to having been assigned tasks for which one is not appropriately trained; and
4. inconsequentiality refers to a feeling that no matter how hard one works, the rewards in terms of accomplishment, recognition, advancement or appreciation are not there.

Preventing Burnout

In order to deal with burnout, the individual must acknowledge its presence. By contrast, it is all too common for those in the health service professions to deny that there is any problem whatsoever. As we can see from the above discussion, one of the problems of burnout is that its symptoms and causes are neither universal to the condition nor specific in nature. This can make it difficult for workers to realize they have burnout.

However, despite this, coping with burnout requires first and foremost a recognition of the problem by the sufferer. There is no point in trying to avoid the problem. Often, becoming aware that one has a potential problem with burnout leads to the belief that it is all one's own fault. There is a sense of shame associated with not being able to cope with work. Becoming aware of the problem is also (one hopes) associated with becoming aware of the cause of the problem. According to Pines *et al.* (1981), it is important that nurses recognize that the problems they face are largely a function of the situation rather than a function of their own dispositional failings.

Taking responsibility for one's own actions is also considered to be important in efforts to deal with burnout. In particular, Pines *et al.* (1981) argue that the professional must be willing to take responsibility for changing the environment if burnout is to be avoided. This may prove difficult for some people who are reluctant to attempt to change their situation, the rationale for this reluctance often being found in their belief that it is the organization's responsibility. Unfortunately, in the nursing profession, as elsewhere, one cannot count on the organization to do anything about problems faced by individual members of staff. The attitude that 'that is the way it has always been in this hospital/ agency and that is the way it will stay' is all too common.

Activities directed towards changing organizational structures are difficult but are worth the effort. Individuals report that they find such efforts to change situations extremely invigorating and therapeutic. The point here is that a single individual within a large organization can often feel lost and alone, but attempting to instigate change can make a difference. In a practical sense, group discussions in which individuals can air concerns could be a good way to start. Work-based support groups are discussed a little later on in this chapter.

One cannot, however, change all aspects of organizational structures, and it would be silly to imagine that one could. It is important to be able to distinguish between those aspects of an organization that cannot be changed and those that can (Pines *et al.*, 1981). For example, one area in which nurses feel frustrated at times relates to the perceived lack of recognition and appreciation they receive from their superiors for the work they do. Instigating some model of peer appreciation in the workplace may be one useful method to counter these negative feelings.

Learning to distinguish between realistic job demands and self-imposed demands is also important. As Pines *et al.* (1981) have pointed out, some in the helping professions regularly overwork, assuming this is a demand placed on them by their organization, but which, if examined more closely, is a self-imposed personal expectation. Nurses (and others in the helping professions) must learn to protect themselves in organizations which place high work demands upon workers, and be able to separate out 'real' demands from 'perceived' demands.

Coping with burnout (or the threat of it) is not easy. A number of strategies have been proposed for managing burnout. In general terms two types of coping have been identified and labelled by the psychologist Lazarus (1966). These are:

1. direct coping, in which the person attempts to deal personally and directly with the source of the stress arising from the situation in which they find themselves; and
2. palliation, in which the person attempts to reduce the personal consequences associated with such external stressors.

Pines *et al.* (1981) have extended this view, suggesting that in addition to the direct/palliative (or in their terminology, direct/indirect) dimensions of coping, their research on burnout in the helping professions reveals an inactive/active dimension. An *active or approach coping strategy* involves confronting or attempting to change the environmental source of the stress or, alternatively, looking to change one's personal perceptions of the situation. By contrast, an *inactive or avoidance coping strategy* involves avoidance of the stressor by withdrawing from it or denying its importance.

As Pines and her colleagues have shown, these two dimensions, direct/indirect and active/inactive, in fact generate four types of coping strategies, each of them represented by three kinds of possible actions:

1. The active/direct form of coping involves change, confrontation or re-evaluation of the source of stress.

2. Those adopting the inactive/direct form attempt to ignore the source of stress, avoid it or leave the situation altogether.
3. Active/indirect copers talk to others about the source of stress, change themselves in order to adapt to it or become involved in other activities to reduce its impact.
4. The use of alcohol or other drugs, developing and manifesting illness or collapsing totally may be seen in those using inactive/indirect strategies.

Pines *et al.* (1981) found that helping professionals who use active coping strategies successfully find that they alleviate distress, because active strategies are likely to change the source of the stress directly. A nurse may seek to change a difficult situation, for example, by confronting her supervisor, or she might attempt to avoid the source of stress, for example, by ignoring the outburst of a patient. She might also seek to resolve her perceptions of the source of her stress indirectly, for example, by talking about it with a friend. Nurses employing each of these (direct) strategies will experience less distress than, say, the nurse who drinks after work to forget the source of her stress.

Apart from these general mechanisms for coping with burnout, there are a number of specific strategies, identified in the literature, which may assist individuals in coping with burnout. Chief among these are the development of work-based support groups, the provision of information/training, the development of self-management strategies, and the development of a state of 'detached concern'.

Development of Work-based Support Groups

Many of the recommendations researchers have made for combating burnout stem directly from research on stress. Maslach, for example, suggests that workers should be advised to form mutual support groups to help them cope with job stress. Support groups have, in fact, been identified as a primary tool in preventing burnout (Scully, 1983). Work-based support groups are one mechanism by which an organization can formally demonstrate its support for staff. It is, if you like, the organization's attempt to offset the occupational stress present in the health services environment.

Support groups are designed to help members deal with stressful work situations. They provide a forum in which members are able to compare and share experiences (Selder & Paustian, 1989). In structure, the support group resembles a discussion group. The goal of the support group is to increase staff feelings of effectiveness and to build a sense of competence, as well as assist staff to feel that they can deal with the stresses they encounter in their work situation. Part of the rationale for support groups is that staff will function more effectively if they can reach a 'psychological middle ground', that is, somewhere between feeling stripped of defences and feeling so defensive that they have no sensitivity whatsoever to those around them. Helping staff find this middle ground is one of the major aims of support groups (Scully, 1983).

The method for reaching this goal is a problem-solving one. In keeping with the consultation nature of the support group, the content of the discussion in such groups must be work related (Scully, 1983). Specifically, staff may discuss in the group whatever work situations may be troubling them, and these are then examined carefully and systematically. Such groups seek to ascertain and discuss questions such as:

- What is the issue?
- Why is this a problem?
- What feelings are associated with the situation?
- What factors contribute to this situation?
- What can be done about the situation?
- What will be the likely consequence of various approaches to solving the problem?
- How will one know when the problem is solved?

As you will recall from discussion earlier in this chapter, the nursing profession has inherent stressors such as patient care, tensions inside the work group, forces outside the work group and unrealistic self-expectations. The support group can provide a mechanism for handling each of these stressors. Let us consider some examples.

Patient Care

The support group can provide a mechanism for dealing with patient-care stressors. Specifically, the group provides a safe place to ventilate feelings of anger, despair, hopelessness, sadness and so on which are often associated with caring for critically ill patients. Once this catharsis has occurred, staff can more realistically examine the source of their feelings. In addition, as staff share their feelings, they realize that they are not alone in the way they are feeling. This sense of togetherness can reassure the individual and also strengthen group bonds. After some of the emotion in the stressful situation has been diffused, the group can search for alternative ways to deal with patient-care stressors.

Tensions Inside the Work Group

Competition for positions of power, interpersonal friction and destructive group norms are all facets of this source of stress. Support groups are able to identify sources of stress by bringing group norms or the unwritten rules of the group to the conscious awareness of the group. After the norms are identified, the support group can clarify the effect that adherence to these unwritten rules may be having on the work group. As a result, the group can examine various alternative mechanisms to meet the needs that the norm was originally established to satisfy.

Forces Outside the Work Group

Low staff numbers, inadequate supplies, poor administrative support or ineffective communication between various levels within an organization can all lead to stress in nurses. The support group helps staff to deal with these stressors by challenging the staff's perceived lack of control of them. While assuming some responsibility for changing these situations can appear daunting at first, efforts to change situations are well worthwhile. A support group can facilitate discussion on immediate and practical ways for dealing with external stressors such as inadequate staffing patterns, handling difficult superiors and gaining administrative support for organizational change.

Unrealistic Self-expectations

Nurses often report that they experience this kind of stress in the form of intense guilt, and in feelings of helplessness and anger. The support group may help staff to deal with these feelings by fostering increased self-awareness. Self-awareness is a crucial step in dealing with unrealistic self-expectations. The support group is able to engender a sense of acceptance and empathy that allows acknowledgement of the threat of unrealistic self-expectations to the nurse's self-concept. Being aware that it is her problem rather than the patient's problem may, for example, help the nurse to set more realistic and attainable goals for her work with patients.

Provision of Information/Training

It is important to recognize that in order to take care of someone else you must first take care of yourself (Yarborough, 1989). Lyall (1989) has noted, for example, that all too often health service workers fail to take adequate psychological care of themselves. He argues that while the fault may lie with the helper, so too does the solution. The provision of adequate information and training may well be a key to ensuring that helpers can take better care of themselves and, by implication, take better care of their patients.

One of the problems identified by researchers working in the area of burnout is the lack of adequate training for nurses concerning the emotional stresses they are likely to experience during the course of their work. Indeed, a large part of the difficulty confronting nurses appears to be the failure of educational programs to teach nurses that they, along with their patients, are likely to suffer emotional stresses. It appears that training programs for health service workers focus on the people receiving the services, with little attention being given to the providers of those services. Gilliland & James (1988) argue that early on in a health service worker's training, and after that on an ongoing basis when in practice, emphasis needs to be placed on the individual worker's attitudes and expectations regarding the profession they have chosen. In-service programs on burnout and stress management programs may be useful in this regard. They particularly note the work of Carroll & White, who have criticized training programs for turning out specialist technicians rather than 'well-rounded' professionals.

For instance, Kramer (1974), in her book *Reality Shock,* has written about the devastating impact which the work of providing a helping service may have on unprepared nurses fresh out of training and new to their careers. One way to decrease uncertainty about what is meant by burnout is to offer 'prophylactic' information to health professionals about the nature of the burnout syndrome and its characteristics, prevention and treatment.

Though health service workers may only be vaguely aware of it at the beginning of their careers, the conflict between externally imposed professional expectations and a person's own idea about the provision of helping services rapidly brings about a need for self-protection. This 'reality shock' most probably results in the documented high turnover rate of nurses in the first few months of their job (Pines *et al.,* 1981). More recently, Randall & Scott (1988) have confirmed that burnout is more likely to occur among newcomers to the profession of nursing than it is among experienced nurses. Early survival in the profession seems, therefore, to bode well for protection against ultimate burnout.

Self-management Strategies

Given the evidence on personal responsibility, training nurses in self-management strategies could prove worthwhile in the treatment and prevention of burnout. Stress management courses, for example, may be distinctly useful in this regard. Self-management strategies increase the feeling of certainty and control over the individual's own well-being (Selder & Paustian, 1989). Used in conjunction with structured relaxation programs (see Chapter 3 for an example of one method of relaxation), self-management strategies have considerable potential in the fight against burnout among nurses.

Developing a State of 'Detached Concern'

The issue of 'detached concern' was raised earlier in this chapter. You will recall that it refers to nurses being sufficiently detached in their attitudes toward the patient to be able exercise sound professional judgement while, at the same time, displaying sensitivity and a level of understanding care toward the patient. Clearly, this optimum balance between over-involvement and depersonalization is difficult to achieve. The establishment of detached concern is really about using the basic therapeutic skills of empathy, unconditional positive regard and congruence (as we have discussed in detail in Chapters 2 and 3). However, to perform in a professionally efficient manner and avoid traumatic problems is quite another matter, and one that requires the nurse to be ever vigilant toward the subtle nuances of the therapeutic moment, which can all too quickly escalate into a fullscale crisis for both her and her patient. Understanding one's own impact on the helping relationship will considerably help the nurse to handle crisis situations as they arise, and ultimately to avoid burnout.

Summary

In this chapter, burnout was defined and its various components delineated. Burnout was seen to be a commonplace consequence of working in the helping professions, and in the profession of nursing in particular. Many critics have dismissed burnout as simply an 'in' topic, or the price one pays for working in people-oriented professions. A number of reasons, however, were given as to why it is important to address burnout in nursing. Among these is the evidence linking the practice of nursing to problems of job productivity, impairment of social and personal relationships, and a variety of psychological and physical health conditions. The symptoms and stages of burnout were also considered. Various strategies for coping with burnout were then described, and both broad intervention strategies and specific coping strategies were discussed. Particular emphasis was given to work-based support groups as tools for preventing burnout in the workplace. It was argued that nurses, as health professionals at risk of burnout, must recognize the potential for burnout in themselves and in the workplace, and direct their attention toward strategies for actively working to avoid this outcome.

Conclusions

Nursing is a critical profession in modern society, directing its activities to the ultimate benefit of humankind. It requires great technical skill, consummate clinical ability, enormous dedication and a seemingly limitless capacity for giving. Many of the qualities the modern nurse requires can be achieved with training, but an equal number of less tangible qualities are often brought into the profession by the people who are to become nurses. As we have shown, these are essentially the characteristics of the person, and as we have gone on to suggest, they form an integral part of the process whereby an individual selects the profession of nursing as the one she will enter. These latter qualities, though they are of undeniable intrinsic value and have much to offer to the practice of nursing, also make the nurse vulnerable to burnout. They may, if unchecked, lead the nurse to expend more effort than she is capable of giving or the organizational and institutional structure of nursing is willing to reward. Most importantly, therefore, this final chapter has been about self-preservation in nursing. If psychology has relevance to the practice of nursing (and the whole substance of this book argues that it does), then it must be put as much to the use of nurses as for the care and well-being of their patients. Nurses are invaluable resources for our society, and their loss through burnout is inexcusable. Burnout is also preventable, however, and we hope that in reading this final chapter, nurses entering this profession will take with them the skills necessary to achieve this effectively.

References/Reading List

Cartwright, L.K. (1979). Sources and effects of stress in health careers. In G.C. Stone, F. Cohen & N.E. Adler (eds), *Health Psychology*. San Francisco: Jossey-Bass Publishers.

Cherniss, C. (1980). *Professional Burnout in Human Service Organizations*. New York: Praegar.

Cherniss, C. & Krantz, D.L. (1983). The ideological community as an antidote to burnout in the human services. In B.A. Farber (ed.), *Stress and Burnout in the Human Service Professions*. New York: Pergamon Press.

Edelwich, J.E. & Brodsky, A. (1980). *Burnout: Stages of Disillusionment in the Helping Professions*. New York: Human Services Press.

Eisenstat, R.A. & Felner, R.D. (1983). Organizational mediators of the quality of care: job stressors and motivators in human service settings. In B.A. Farber (ed.), *Stress and Burnout in the Human Service Professions*. New York: Pergamon Press.

Farber, B.A. (ed.) (1983a). *Stress and Burnout in the Human Service Professions*. New York: Pergamon Press.

Farber, B.A. (1983b). A critical perspective on burnout. In B.A. Farber (ed.), *Stress and Burnout in the Human Service Professions*. New York: Pergamon Press.

Freudenberger, H.J. (1974). Staff burnout. *Journal of Social Issues*, 30, 159–165.

Freudenberger, H.J. (1975). The staff burn-out syndrome in alternative institutions. *Psychotherapy: Theory, Research and Practice*, 12, 73–82.

Freudenberger, H.J. (1983). Burnout: contemporary issues, trends, and concerns. In B.A. Farber (ed.), *Stress and Burnout in the Human*

Service Professions. New York: Pergamon Press.

Freudenberger, H.J. (1989). An overview of burnout. In D.T. Wessells *et al.* (eds), *Professional Burnout in Medicine and the Helping Professions.* New York: The Haworth Press.

Freudenberger, H.J. & Richelson, G. (1980). *Burn-out: The High Cost of High Achievement.* New York: Anchor Press.

Gilliland, B.E. & James, R.K. (1988). *Crisis Intervention Strategies.* Pacific Grove, California: Brooks/Cole.

Golembiewski, R.T., Munzenrider, R.F. & Stevenson, J.G. (1986). *Stress in Organizations: Toward a Phase Model of Burnout.* New York: Praeger.

Heifetz, L.J. & Bersani, H.A. (1983). Disrupting the cybernetics of personal growth: toward a unified theory of burnout in the human services. In B.A. Farber (ed.), *Stress and Burnout in the Human Service Professions.* New York: Pergamon Press.

Jayaratne, S. & Chess, W.A. (1983). Job satisfaction and burnout in social work. In B.A. Farber (ed.), *Stress and Burnout in the Human Service Professions.* New York: Pergamon Press.

Jones, J.W. (ed.) (1982). *The Burnout Syndrome. Current Research, Theory, Interventions.* Park Ridge, Illinois: London House Press.

Kramer, M. (1974). *Reality Shock.* St Louis: C.V. Mosby Company.

Lazarus, R.S. (1966). *Psychological Stress and the Coping Process.* New York: McGraw-Hill.

Lyall, R. (1989). Burnout in the professional care giver: does the phoenix have to burn or why can't Icarus stay aloft? In D.T. Wessells *et al.* (eds), *Professional Burnout in Medicine and the Helping Professions.* New York: The Haworth Press.

McConnell, E.A. (1982). *Burnout in the Nursing Profession: Coping Strategies, Causes and Costs.* St Louis: C.V. Mosby Company.

Maslach, C. (1976). Burned out. *Human Behavior,* 5, 16–22.

Maslach, C. (1978). The client role in staff burn-out. *Journal of Social Issues,* 34, 111–123.

Maslach, C. (1982). *Burnout: The Cost of Caring.* Englewood Cliffs, New Jersey: Prentice-Hall.

Maslach, C. & Jackson, S.E. (1981). The measurement of experienced burnout. *Journal of Occupational Behavior,* 2, 99–113.

Maslach, C. & Jackson, S.E. (1982). Burnout in health professions: a social psychological analysis. In G. Sanders & J. Suls (eds), *Social Psychology of Health and Illness.* Hillsdale, New Jersey: Erlbaum.

Maslach, C. & Pines, A. (1979). 'Burnout', the loss of human caring. In A. Pines & C. Maslach (eds), *Experiencing Social Psychology.* New York: Random House.

Meier, S.T. (1983). Toward a theory of burnout. *Human Relations,* 36, 899–910.

Paine, W.S. (1982). Overview of burnout stress syndromes and the 1980's. In W.S. Paine (ed.), *Job Stress and Burnout.* Beverly Hills, California: Sage Publications.

Patterson, C.H. (1980). *Theories of Counselling and Psychotherapy.* New York: Harper & Row.

Pines, A. (1983). On burnout and the buffering effects of social support. In B.A. Farber (ed.), *Stress and Burnout in the Human Service Professions.* New York: Pergamon Press.

Pines, A., Aronson, E. & Kafry, D. (1981). *Burnout: From Tedium to Personal Growth.* New York: Free Press.

Pines, A. & Maslach, C. (1978). Characteristics of staff burnout in mental health settings. *Hospital and Community Psychiatry,* 29, 233–237.

Randall, M. & Scott W.A. (1988). Burnout, job satisfaction, and job performance. *Australian Psychologist,* 23, 335–347.

Riggar, T.F., Harrington, G.S. & Hafer, M. (1984). Burnout and job satisfaction in rehabilitation administrators and direct service providers. *Rehabilitation Counselling Bulletin,* 27, 151–160.

Scully, R. (1983). The work-setting support group: a means of preventing burnout. In B.A. Farber (ed.), *Stress and Burnout in the Human Service Professions.* New York: Pergamon Press.

Selder, F.E. & Paustian, A. (1989). Burnout: absence of vision. In D.T. Wessells *et al.* (eds), *Professional Burnout in Medicine and the Helping Professions.* New York: The Haworth Press.

Weiner, W. (1989). Is burnout an institutional syndrome? In D.T. Wessells *et al.* (eds), *Professional Burnout in Medicine and the Helping Professions.* New York: The Haworth Press.

Wessells, D.T., Kutscher, A.H., Seeland, I.B., Selder, F.E., Cherico, D.J. & Clarke, E.J. (eds) (1989). *Professional Burnout in Medicine and the Helping Professions.* New York: The Haworth Press.

Yarborough, T.E. (1989). A day with our feelings. In D.T. Wessells *et al.* (eds), *Professional Burnout in Medicine and the Helping Professions.* New York: The Haworth Press.

Index